C000151763

This book is dedicated to my dear friend, Kaye Falconer, who has not only been my guinea pig and biohacking partner in crime for the past 6 years, but has encouraged me almost every time we met to write this book.

Health Disclaimer

The information in this e-book is for general information purposes and nothing contained in it is, or is intended to be construed as advice. It does not take into account your individual health, medical, physical or emotional situation or needs. It is not a substitute for medical attention, treatment, examination, advice, treatment of existing conditions or diagnosis and is not intended to provide a clinical diagnosis nor take the place of proper medical advice from a fully qualified medical practitioner. You should, before you act or use any of this information, consider the appropriateness of this information having regard to your own personal situation and needs. You are responsible for consulting a suitable medical professional before using any of the information or materials contained in this book.

Copyright © 2020 Lynn Hardy

You may not share, copy or redistribute this Material in any medium or format at any time. Our materials are for your individual personal use only and may not be used for commercial purposes. You are not permitted to make any derivative material, including but not limited to copying, reproducing, transforming, sharing or building upon the material in whole or any part thereof. For any other use or distribution, you must have express written consent from the author.

THE
Aging Games

HOW TO COME OUT A WINNER

Over 100 Anti-aging tips

*By **Lynn Hardy, ND, CNC***

Table of Contents

CHAPTER 7

Spa & Medical Treatments

CHAPTER 8

Additional Links & Resources

Introduction

I have been involved in the natural health industry for almost 30 years and have found there are very natural and effective ways to feel and look young as we enter our more mature years. Once I turned 50, I realized that 50 may be the new 30, and 50 is a very beautiful and sexy age to be. The world looks at us differently today, thanks to the many youthful older celebrities that grace our televisions screens and also with women in general taking better care of themselves.

With that being said, I also want people to know you don't have to spend like a celebrity to feel and look your best. There are so many things you can do at home every day to keep yourself young and healthy; and if you don't feel young and healthy, you soon can, with a little work.

The key is discipline and persistence. Many of the hacks I include in this book are easy to implement at home, and while they may not seem like much on their own, they add up to big changes. There are over 100 hacks included under "solutions" in each topic. If you choose 20 of them and do your best to implement them on most days, you will see and feel a difference. I promise!

The more you do, the quicker you will see results. No matter if you are 40, 50, 60 or 70 and beyond, I believe you can help your body and mind become healthier. The key is to not stress or beat yourself up if you cannot follow or do all of these age-hacking ideas. For example, I include a lot of information about diet, but if you have been eating sweets or high-sugar foods for a long time, you may not be able to give those up right away.

Don't try to change overnight. Instead, try incorporating small and persistent changes at first. If you want to give up sugar, then cut it out for one or two days a week and build from there. Your taste buds will change, and you will get used to it. Treat each challenge like this and you will be like the turtle from Aesop's fables and win; here it isn't a race, but the Aging Games.

Please keep in mind that these hacks are based on my own personal research and experience. You will definitely not agree with everything, and all tips are not for everybody. Please don't take it personally if we have different opinions on things. If you've found a diet, exercise program or beauty hacks that work for you, then by all means, please continue to do them. If you suffer from any health conditions, please do check with your doctor before making any changes or implementing anything recommended in these pages.

I hope you do enjoy this book and learn a few new things. You may choose to keep it on hand and use it as a reference. Try out 10 hacks, and if you like, add 10 more in a month, or change to an entirely different 10 hacks. You can also try one from each category to start with. The choice is yours, and the best way to go about it is to relax and enjoy the journey. And with that, I say…

Let the Games Begin

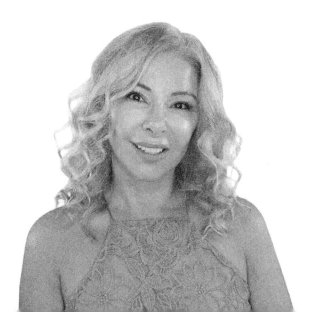

CHAPTER 1

Home Practices

I'm going to begin with home practices because these are easy hacks to implement. And while they just seem like "things you do," it is small things like these that can make a big difference. Since most of these are easy to incorporate into your everyday life, along with instructing how to do each hack, I will inform you of why you should try them out. I find that many times, when my students and clients know why a certain act is performed, it adds motivation to actually doing it. I hope you find these interesting and helpful.

Cleaning Products and Their Impact on Your Health

Eliminate toxic cleaning products and similar items in your environment. Our culture is very engrained into using bleach, disinfectants and other harsh chemicals to make sure all bacteria, germs and/or pathogens are knocked out dead in their tracks. Unfortunately, some ingredients in these products are actually harmful to our health. They can confuse our immune system and cause harmful bacteria (and other harmful microbes) to mutate, allowing them to become stronger. Also keep in mind that our bodies contain about 39 trillion microorganisms and bacteria, without which we would not exist, therefore killing bacteria should not always be the end-goal.

The harsh chemicals found in everyday cleaning products can also interfere with our natural immunity by overstimulating our immune systems or interfering with healthy hormonal activity; and as we age, the effects of this become even more apparent and harmful. First, let's take a look at some chemicals and their harmful effects they may have on health, according to the Environmental Working Group:[1]

---

1   Cleaning Supplies and Your Health. (n. d.). Retrieved October 21, 2020, from https://www.ewg.org/guides/cleaners/content/cleaners_and_health/

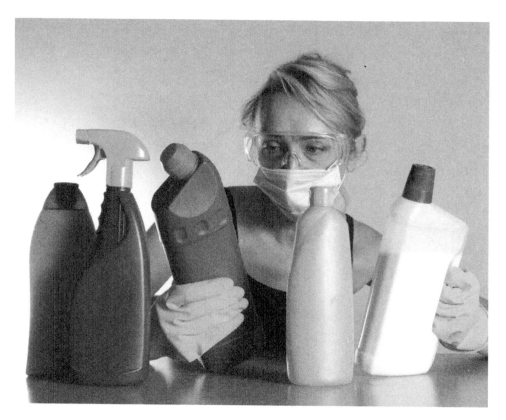

- Poisoning and chemical burns are the more obvious effects, and products like these often come with warnings. If you must use them, do not be in a closed room while using them and limit your exposure.

- In high amounts, Borax and boric acid, often used as an ingredient in laundry and dishwashing detergents, are linked to issues with the sex organs, problems like testicular atrophy in males and reduced fertility in females. Worse, they have the ability to cross over into the placenta of a pregnant woman and affect birth weight and fetal skeletal development.

- Studies show that nearly one in three cleaning workers develop atopic dermatitis.

- Common or ordinary cleaning of office, workspaces, schools and other public spaces releases volatile fumes within minutes of use, which can travel through the air or ventilation system. Fumes such as ammonia and glycol ether have been linked to increased asthma, eczema and allergies.

- Fragrances are a top allergen and about one in five people who are exposed to them suffer breathing difficulties and headaches, while one study found that home air fresheners are linked to depression in adults as well as earaches and diarrhea in infants (Farrow 2003).

- Chlorine and phosphoric acids are commonly used in cleaning products and can lead to cell dehydration and interfere with natural hormonal action as they affect the thyroid. As we age, the organs become more fragile and the need to take care of them becomes more important. Anyone who has experienced low thyroid with age is familiar with symptoms that seem to be associated with premature aging, including frizzy hair and unexplained weight gain.

Cleaning ingredients vary in the type of health hazard they produce. Some cause acute, or immediate issues such as skin or respiratory irritation, watery eyes, or chemical burns, while others are associated with chronic, or long-term, effects such as cancer.

✓The Solution

So, what can we use to clean our homes? The first simple solution is to find products labeled as "non-toxic" and then read the ingredients. Not all labels are honest, as they may add a mystery "fragrance" or unnamed "natural ingredients." Many ingredients can be named natural if they are found in nature, but it doesn't mean we should inhale or interact with them.

Making your own cleaners is another option. While that would take an entire chapter for a list of how to make safe cleaners, the following will give you an idea of how it's done:

- A handful of citrus peels through the garbage disposal will safely clean any smells from the sink.

- Stainless steel, including sinks and cookware, can be cleaned with olive oil and undiluted white vinegar. Follow with a baking soda scrub to rinse and complete cleaning.

- Make your own toilet bowl cleaner with ¼ cup baking soda and 1 cup of vinegar, pour into the toilet basin, allow it to set for a few minutes, then scrub with your toilet bowl brush.

- Tub and tile can be cleaned with baking soda, using water to dampen it, or wipe surface with vinegar first for tougher jobs.

- Window cleaner can be made with 2 teaspoons of white vinegar to one quart of water. Use a cotton cloth to apply and clean your windows.

As you can see, there are many household products that are used, and each one has potentially harmful chemicals. While one product, once in a while may not be that bad, toxins from product use accumulates, which are the culprits that can overwhelm your organs, disrupt your hormones and cause premature aging and various illnesses.

Home Lighting and Blue Light Elimination

Limit all blue light at night so you can get a good night's sleep. Sleep is important for all generations, especially mature adults. When you cannot sleep well, your entire life will be impacted, including being at a higher risk for accidents or falls, memory issues, irritability and depression. While I will cover why optimal sleep is important later, the lighting you use in your home before sleep is also crucial.

Blue light waves are found everywhere in our environment. We are surrounded by both natural blue light and artificial blue light, and while the beautiful color blue is often associated with calm and healing, an abundance of artificial blue light exposure can cause problems like headaches, fatigue, eyestrain and vision problems as well as insomnia. Blue light is a melatonin suppressant, and melatonin is a crucial hormone for healthy sleep.

It is ideal to get sunshine every day, and that used to be our main exposure of blue light, however with the sun, blue light does not appear in isolation. Natural blue light helps the body form a healthy circadian rhythm that supports our natural sleep cycle. But today, we have brought artificial blue light inside our homes, through televisions, Smartphones, and computers.

Artificial blue light interferes with our natural circadian rhythm as it tricks the brain into believing that day is day and night is day, as well. The problem has scientists and medical experts very concerned as the interruption of our natural sleep may be behind an increased risk for health issues like diabetes, heart disease and cancer. Exposure to blue light before sleep every night can actually raise your blood sugar and insulin levels as if you were diabetic. This can happen even on a very low-carb diet.

Unlike the chronic, low-level blue light exposure that affects the brain, blue light therapy devices using short-term, targeted energy are not considered harmful, and are used in beauty salons or at home to treat acne, reduce inflammation and improve skin's texture.

✓ The Solution

There is an array of solutions to replace or tone down blue light use in your home. Some fun alternatives are to use candles. The right candles not only make your home feel warm and cozy, but you can use them as regular light and even to read at night. Use organic candles with natural scents to avoid inhaling toxic fumes. Other solutions include:

- Stick to natural light to light your home as often as possible during the day

- Use alternative lightbulbs in your home such as warm, low-wattage red nightlights and yellow lights

- Install blue light blocking software on computers, laptops, and phones

- Wear blue light blocking glasses, especially when using your phone or laptop at night

- Install blue light screen filters on all monitors, LED displays and phones

- Sleep with an eye mask

- Read from real books at night before bed, instead of watching TV or browsing on your phone

- Remove light pollution from glowing electronic devices by covering them or simply removing them from the room, especially your sleeping area

Healthy Sun Exposure

We are all taught that exposure to the sun will lead to skin cancer, hyperpigmentation, and premature wrinkles. Because of this, many people flood to the outdoors covered in toxic sunscreen, hoping to protect their skin from the horrors of the sun's harmful UVB radiation. But there is much more to sunshine and the sunscreen that you should be aware of.

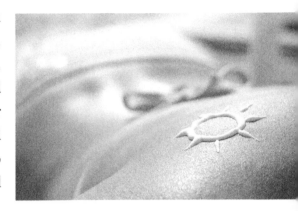

Sunlight is a necessary component the body needs to make vitamin D, which helps strengthen bones and muscles, boosts your immune system and protects you from just about every type of cancer. While you can get some Vitamin D through food, current research is showing that deficiencies of vitamin D are mainly due to lack of sun exposure.[2]

But we need sun for more than just this important vitamin. We need it to improve our moods, because sunlight seems to have a direct impact on serotonin levels, a hormone that helps you feel happy. In fact, many people who live in wintery areas are well aware of Seasonal Affective Disorder (SAD), which is a form of depression that comes about with overcast, wintery skies (symptoms often begin in late fall and last until spring).

Getting a healthy dose of sunshine is also known to help you sleep better, make you feel happier, helps with weight maintenance, strengthens your immune system and helps ward off depression. And a look at the cumulative data shows that lack of sun creates a much greater health burden and is linked to numerous diseases worldwide. One example is that skin

2   Mead MN. Benefits of sunlight: a bright spot for human health [published correction appears in Environ Health Perspect. 2008 May; 116(5):A197]. Environ Health Perspect. 2008;116(4):A160-A167. doi:10.1289/ehp.116-a160

cancer is associated with too much sun exposure, but too little sun exposure increases the risk of other types of cancers including ovarian, colon and breast cancer![3]

But is the sun really to blame for skin cancer, or is it caused by toxic sunscreens and the overuse of vegetable oils in our diet? Dr. Jack Kruse, a famous neurosurgeon in the biohacking community, has thousands of followers and the consensus is always the same. Once people stop using vegetable oils for cooking, their skin no longer burns in the sun and they can finally get a beautiful, healthy tan, like never before.

The longer I live the more beautiful life becomes.

—**Frank Lloyd Wright**

Most of us have been indoctrinated to slather large amounts of sunscreen all over the body, every time we go outside. It is only recently that scientists are finding at least five of the toxic ingredients absorb into the skin and remain in the body indefinitely. In fact, two of the chemicals, oxybenzone and octinoxate, are responsible for killing off coral, possibly from so many sunscreen drenched bodies swimming in the water.

Some scientists and/or doctors claim we should not be worried about the potential toxic effects of sunscreens but keep in mind this is a huge industry, as is the pharmaceutical industry, which profits from the illnesses caused by lack of sunlight and overuse of toxins. If the sun was truly out to eliminate humankind, we would have died out a long time ago.

Just think back to our childhood. Most have never even heard of skin cancer, much less known someone who had it. We also didn't use sunscreen and happily baked in the sun all summer. So what changed since then?

---

3   Mead MN. Benefits of sunlight: a bright spot for human health [published correction appears in Environ Health Perspect. 2008 May;116(5):A197]. Environ Health Perspect. 2008;116(4):A160-A167. doi:10.1289/ehp.116-a160

Was it the sun, or something else that we're doing? Food for thought, right?

I believe it is better to be proactive and take our life into our own hands. Keeping harmful chemicals out of your bloodstream is a first step, and important to prolonging your life, and there are alternatives. As for sun aging your skin, obviously you don't need too much of a good thing. But let's take a closer look at what can be done.

There is a fountain of youth: it is your mind, your talents, the creativity you bring to your life and the lives of people you love. When you learn to tap this source, you will truly have defeated age.

—Sophia Loren

✓The Solution:

Do you need to wear sunscreen? According to Dr. Kruse, not if you spend enough time exposing your skin to the sun's rays in the early morning and late afternoon before sundown. During those times there are no UV rays present and the infrared rays will prepare your skin for the coming UV rays around solar noon.

Infrared light is the sunscreen we need to protect us from the deleterious effects of UV radiation. Do you see how brilliant nature is? Once you've built your sun callus, you can safely expose your skin to high UV rays during midday for optimal Vitamin D production. In the afternoon, as the sun begins to set, the infrared rays will help repair any damage to skin that has been overexposed to UV rays during the day.

The takeaway? According to Dr. Kruse, "If you are going to the beach this summer, get there EARLY, stay LATER, and make sure your skin is exposed to lots of early mornings and late afternoon sunshine! During solar noon, get enough sun so that your skin gets flush but does not burn. Then wear clothing and hats to block the sun's rays until late afternoon

> *"Your solar callus not only offers protection, but it is an ideal way to absorb sunlight properly to get light into your system to build wellness and improve your immunity. Our skin tones are tied to our solar callus and are perceived as most healthy and attractive to humans. We know that red and yellow skin tones make you appear more attractive and send wireless signals to others that your immune system is optimized. Being pale is not a sign of wellness contrary to popular dermatologic speeches. Even animals besides humans use their solar callus to draw mates."*
>
> **Dr. Jack Kruse**

and then... get naked again! The more exposure you give your skin to early morning sunlight, the more resilient it will be to the UV rays midday."

So what can you do to safely protect yourself from too much exposure? Of course, the obvious thing is to cover up or stay in the shade once you've reached your optimal exposure time. There is also the option of using non-toxic sunscreens which are available as a healthier alternative to the standard products sold commercially. Non-toxic sunscreens are made with the minerals such as zinc or titanium dioxide or a combination of both. Be wary of those that are simply labeled as "mineral based," because these often include one or both of these minerals along with the standard, chemical sunscreens.

Other Home Practices–Your Personal Environment

Reduce Cell Phone Radiation

Cell phones emit an energy called non-ionizing radiation. While there are still many skeptics that believe this type of low-level energy is not harmful, many experts now claim there is a link between cell phone radiation and cancer and other diseases. Dr. Jack Kruse, neurosurgeon, has spoken out about how he's seeing glioblastoma (the deadliest form of brain cancer) in younger and younger patients in his practice. He attributes this alarming trend to cell phone radiation. A new study published in Clinical Neurophysiology suggests it doesn't take years or even months of exposure for cell phone radiation to negatively alter our brains—it only takes minutes.

Repeated exposure to radiation will cause damage to your skin, immune system and internal organs, leading to premature aging, disease and early death.

But it doesn't end there. Other issues to worry about with cell phone exposure are materials used in the cell phone cases. For example, nickel and chromium are often used and also known to stimulate allergic skin issues like dermatitis. Additionally, most mobile phones emit blue light, which was already discussed above. But don't worry, this doesn't mean you have to break up with your cell phone for good.

✓ The Solution

The first and most obvious is to use your phone only when absolutely necessary. For scrolling and searching the internet, it is much better and safer to use a wired computer.

When you are speaking on your phone, keep it at least three inches from your ear or better yet, use the speaker phone or RF safe headsets. Texting is also a safer option. You should also pay attention to where your phone is stored. For example, I can't help but cringe when women carry their phones in their bras or men with phones in their pockets, next to their genitals.

Other precautions to take are using an anti-radiation phone case, which can block radiation and protect you, especially if you keep your phone in your pocket. Anti-radiation headsets can be used that have both speakers and a microphone, so the phone doesn't have to be close to your head at

Wearing a cell phone on your hip—either on your belt or in a pocket—has been linked to decreased bone density in the pelvic region. All the other vital organs located in your pelvic region—your liver, kidney, bladder, colon and reproductive organs—are also susceptible to radiation damage.

all. Lastly, avoid talking on your phone if you have a weak signal, since the phone reacts by boosting radiofrequency transmission power.

Reduce Wi-Fi Exposure

Wireless technologies have allowed us far greater freedom to roam about our homes and in public while using our phones, searching the internet and even watching television. But just like cell phones, research shows that Wi-Fi affects our health in a very negative way.

Wi-Fi is a wireless network that involves at least one Wi-Fi antenna, often used to connect to wireless devices to the internet. Considered a form of microwave frequency, Wi-Fi is becoming more of a cause for health concerns. Some studies are linking it to oxidative stress, which is a state in which the immune system does not have enough antioxidants to combat free radicals. This lowers the immune response and can accelerate the aging process.

Other effects from Wi-Fi exposure may include DNA damage to cells, endocrine changes, and apoptosis (cell death) of healthy cells. The brain, heart and testis are the organs most sensitive to damage.

I would prefer to not turn this into a discussion about whether these claims are based in science or merely anecdotal evidence, but you can find 23 controlled, scientific

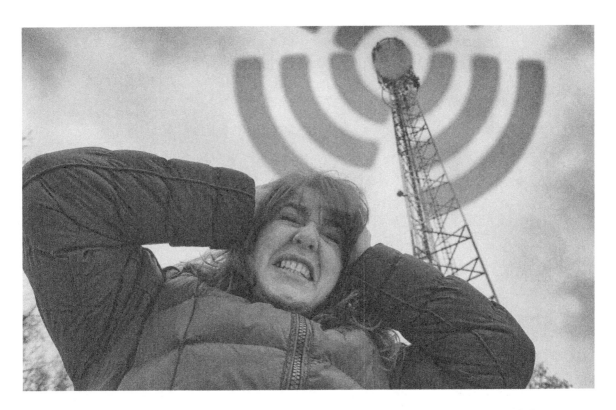

studies on the effects of Wi-Fi on rats, human cells in a culture and the human body on the ScienceDirect website.[4]

✓ The Solution

Reducing your exposure to Wi-Fi may not always be your choice. But you can start at home with simple steps such as these:

- Do not sleep with your cell phone. Research shows that even having your mobile phone near your bed while you sleep can interrupt normal sleep patterns, even if you're not looking at it. Try putting it across the room, and if you do keep it near you, put the phone on airplane mode.

---

4 Pall, Martin L. "Wi-Fi Is an Important Threat to Human Health." Environmental Research, Academic Press, 21 Mar. 2018, www.sciencedirect.com/science/article/pii/S0013935118300355.

Excessive Wi-Fi exposure is associated with impaired memory, sleep disturbances, and fatigue related to reduced melatonin and increased norepinephrine secretion at night.

- Hardwire your home internet connection; you will also benefit with better internet service.

- Do not wear your phone on your body.

- Do not use an iPad or laptop on your lap; use a table instead as these emit strong radiation. Also keep these devices out of the bedroom or on airplane mode.

- If you must have Wi-Fi in your home, place a timer on the router so that it's not running at night while the family's sleeping.

LED and Fluorescent Lighting

I already covered blue lighting, but need to point out here that LED and fluorescent lighting also have a negative impact on our health. So, what makes them so unhealthy?

I will begin with LED lights, because these are being touted by energy companies and governments alike to replace all your home lighting with LED bulbs. LED stands for light-emitting diode, and these bulbs are considered the future of lighting. They use less energy and can help keep your electric bills down. Today, they are sold as lightbulbs, Christmas or holiday lighting and some energy companies give them away.

The dark side is that LED lights are designed with toxic metals that are hazardous to your health. Some examples are the "low-intensity red LEDs," which contain up to eight times the neurotoxin, lead. In fact, some researchers warn about these lights as they have high amounts of arsenic, as well. Other metals that might be found in any color LED lights are copper and nickel, which can cause allergic reactions. If you have them in your home and it breaks, be sure to take precautions and wear a mask and gloves to clean it up.

Fluorescent lighting emits ultraviolet radiation and increases your exposure to carcinogenic radiation (the kind that causes cancer) by up to 30%. But the problem is not only the radiation, but the quality of light that is emitted. Apparently, the type of light these bulbs throw off disturbs our natural body rhythms and can have side effects such as insomnia, hormonal disruption, eyestrain, stress and anxiety, tumor formation and obesity. But if you must be around either of these lights, you can be proactive and protect yourself.

According to French health authorities, the blue light in LED lighting can damage the eye's retina while disturbing our biological and sleep rhythms.

√The Solution

• Use natural light inside your home and at work as much as possible.

• To counter the effects of lighting, get more sunshine. Natural sunshine will have a positive impact on your health that can strengthen your circadian rhythm.

• If you work in an environment with fluorescent lights, consider asking your boss or the "powers that be" if the lighting is either full spectrum or daylight spectrum (both are better alternatives), and if not, try to request a full spectrum light filter for your area.

LED and fluorescent lights bombard our skin with blue light. According to recent studies, blue light causes skin damage and premature skin aging.

- Replace any flickering fluorescent light bulbs, as these are linked to anxiety and eye strain. If you cannot get away from a flickering bulb, keep an incandescent light bulb on your desk.

- Pick up a pair of very light rose-colored tinted glasses, as these are often prescribed by optometrists to counter fluorescent light effects.

- Change your bulbs at home to incandescent bulbs. These are the old-fashioned bulbs that many of us grew up with. They're not very energy efficient and they don't last long, but your health is much more important.

Optimal Sleep

The next few sections are devoted to helping you get a good night's sleep. Sleep is important through our entire life. Not getting enough sleep will become more apparent as we age. That's because lack of sleep or poor-quality sleep can lead to cognitive problems, confusion, forgetfulness, and a host of other problems that can make you feel older than your age. Poor sleep will also show up on our faces as puffiness, deep lines and lack of luster.

Low-quality sleep can cause one to stay in bed too long, creating physical problems like edema, back and hip pain and more fatigue. Not getting a good night's rest can also make you clumsier during the day, which will increase your chance of accidents and falls; something that should be avoided at all costs when we are older. The following habits can help you practice getting a good night's sleep, and as they say, practice makes perfect.

Sleep Position

Sleep on your back for the myriad of health benefits it provides. We spend roughly one third of our lives lying down and sleeping. We know that sleeping is good for us, both physically and mentally, and there's a reason why the term "beauty sleep" has been a popular expression since at least the 1800s. But why is sleep position so important?

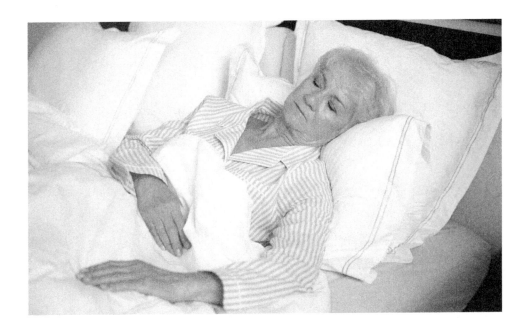

- **Less Facial Wrinkles**—This is the number one reason why so many dermatologists want their patients to sleep on their backs. Sleeping on your side or on your tummy leaves your face scrunched in an un-natural position on your pillow. The result is more pooling of fluids around the eyes and wrinkles that some call sleep lines. These lines form mainly around the mouth, the lateral cheek area, around the eyes and as vertical lines on the forehead. But training yourself to sleep on your back will prevent your face from rubbing on the pillow or mattress, which can not only prevent wrinkles, but help prevent face asymmetry; a condition of uneven face volume and skin texture that dermatologists see when one has a habit of sleeping on their side.

- **Smoother Neck**—The neck is prone to wrinkles just like the face, and we all know that a wrinkled neck can not only show age, but cause one to appear older than they are. Sleeping on your back will prevent the skin on your neck and chin from scrunching and extending to the side, which can lead to an aged look.

- **Smoother Cleavage** - If you sleep on your side, the chest skin will begin to wrinkle. Though you may not realize it initially, over time, you'll get vertical lines in your cleavage, which will thin out the skin.

- **Alleviate Back and Neck Pain**—Sleeping on your back can distribute weight more evenly across your muscles and skeletal system. But sleeping on your side, over time, can cause shoulder and neck pain as your bones are compressed and remain as such throughout the night. Sleeping on your back can also alleviate pressure from your lower back, especially if you keep a pillow under your knees for a healthy spine position that can be maintained through the night without issues.

Sleep Apnea is a problem for some, and for those who suffer, sleeping flat on your back may come with health risks. Sleep apnea is a sleeping disorder where breathing comes to an abrupt halt due to obstructions in the breathing passageway, such as when the throat muscles or sinus muscles relax too much. The sudden feeling of asphyxiation may cause one to constantly wake up during the night, leading to excessive daytime fatigue.

If you suffer from this condition, there are a number of things to try from losing weight to quitting smoking. If you have sleep apnea and you still want to try sleeping on your back, elevate your shoulders and head. Sleeping on an inclined bed can also offer relief from this difficult condition, but more on this later. Also, talk to your doctor as there may be other ways to alleviate the condition, since the cause for each person is often different.

In the central place of every heart there is a recording chamber. So long as it receives a message of beauty, hope, cheer, and courage – so long are you young. When the wires are all down and our heart is covered with the snow of pessimism and the ice of cynicism, then, and only then, are you grown old.

—Douglas MacArthur

Despite all these positive aspects of sleeping on one's back, every theory has at least two sides. According to researchers at Stony Brook University, sleeping in the side position, as compared to sleeping on one's back or stomach, may more effectively remove brain waste and prove to be an important practice to help reduce the chances of developing Alzheimer's, Parkinson's and other neurological diseases. I do believe, as you will see further into the book, that sleeping on an incline can also have similar positive effects, even if you're sleeping on your back.

✓ The Solution

While sleeping on your back may seem like the solution, it is not that easy for many people to go from what they have been comfortable with all their lives to this new position. It may take a little practice, but it's well worth the effort.

- Try elevating your head on a few pillows and then remove a pillow each time you get used to the position. When you get down to one pillow, try to find the height that doesn't leave your neck too crooked, with your chin scrunched into your chest.

- Try supporting pillows on each side of your waist to stop you from naturally rolling over in your sleep. When you wake up in the night sleeping on your side or tummy, simply go back to the supine position.

- Try relaxing your body part-by-part, beginning with your feet and working your way up to your head. This meditation/relaxation technique works wonders for many people.

- Raise the head of your bed 6 inches with bricks or wooden slabs.

Please check out my video about back sleeping:

Channel: The Aging Games
How to sleep on your back | Trying to Train Myself

Also see my video about Inclined Bed Therapy:

Channel: The Aging Games
Inclined Bed Therapy Benefits and Review

Silk Bedding for Anti-Aging and Comfort

Silk bedding has been promoted since the times of Cleopatra for getting a true beauty sleep. And while it seems that the luxury can comfort and soothe you, there are some real, physical reasons to use silk, especially as a tool for anti-aging.

Cotton and linen materials, often used for pillowcases and other bedding, can tug and pull on your skin as you move around through the night. But silk is more forgiving and allows your face to glide over the smooth surface. So, even if you are practicing sleeping on your back, silk will help for those times when you unconsciously roll around through the night.

Silk has benefits for your hair, as well. Silk can help prevent hair breakage and result in less frizzy hair. At the same time, some hair professionals claim that silk allows professional blowouts to last longer.

Anecdotal evidence seems to be the main reason why silk pillowcases and other bedding are so popular. Many people feel when they use a silk pillowcase, they wake up with their hair and face both appearing more refreshed. This may be because cotton and linen can draw moisture out of hair and skin, leaving dryness and irritation. At the same time, slathering your face in moisture cream can cause it to remain on your cotton or linen bedding, also leading to clogged pores as well as dryness, both of which are problems with aging skin.

✓ The Solution

Protect or improve your skin and hair by using a silk pillowcase. The concept is so popular, you can literally perform an internet search with the term, "antiaging silk pillowcase" and find thousands of hits online. With benefits such as preventing crow's feet, lessening forehead wrinkles and elimination of hair frizz and tangling, it's surprising

---

Benefits of silk pillowcases:

- *Less friction on skin or hair prevents irritation or damage.*
- *A cleaner sleep surface.*
- *Less drying for skin and hair.*

that the cost remains low for most brands. Of course, if you want full body antiaging protection, look for an entire silk bedding set.

Inclined Bed Therapy

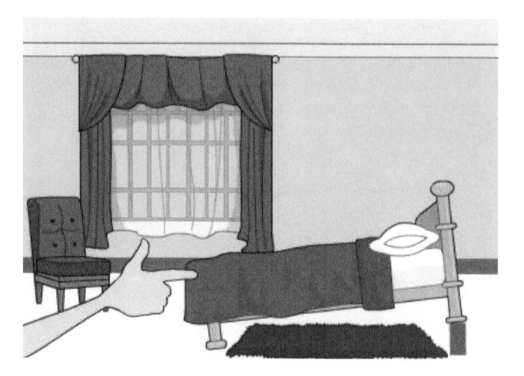

I already discussed the importance of sleep and the importance of sleep position, earlier. I have reserved Inclined Bed Therapy for its own section because it can really add to one's overall health and wellbeing. This is a longstanding practice that has science to back it up, and interestingly, some archeologists believe there is evidence that the ancient Egyptians practiced this way of sleeping.

Inclined Bed Therapy is sleeping on a bed, with the head of the bed lifted 6 inches (15cm) leading to a constant incline of around 5%. The result is that you sleep with your head higher than the rest of your body, which comes with incredible benefits like improved metabolism and circulation.

More importantly, you can enjoy better brain health when sleeping on an incline, which many of us know becomes more important as we age. During sleep, the brain becomes awash with cerebrospinal fluids that help remove heavy metals, pathogens, and other debris. Called the glymphatic system, the brain relies on this fluid to remove waste as well as the removal of blood in exchange for fresh, oxygen and nutrient rich blood while we sleep.

Lying flat as you sleep slows the circulation of cerebrospinal fluid, adding pressure to the inside of the skull. Some doctors believe this lack of drainage may contribute to Alzheimer's disease and other age-related problems as old protein and other debris build up in the brain instead of being rinsed out with the fluid.

Benefits of Inclined Bed Therapy include clearer sinuses, less eye and face puffiness upon awakening, fewer headaches and migraines, improved memory, and lower blood pressure. Other benefits reported that are directly related to sleep position include less snoring and lower incidents of sleep apnea, which allow the brain to get more oxygen through the night.

When we consider how our bodies function through the night, these benefits make sense. And the best part is you don't need any special equipment or bed to try it.

For the unlearned, old age is winter; for the learned, it is the season of the harvest.

—Hasidic saying

When we are inclined in bed, no matter which position we sleep in, gravity is positively acting upon the digestive system by helping to move food more quickly, which helps to prevent constipation or diarrhea.

✓The Solution

To try Inclined Bed Therapy yourself, simply lift the head of your bed by 3.5 to 6 inches. Some people use books, bricks or blocks of wood, but you can also purchase bed risers that are non slip and fit under the feet of the bed.

Keep in mind that inclined bed therapy is not the same as raising the head of your bed with extra pillows or by adjusting the top part of an adjustable bed. The entire bed should be at an incline, ideally at 5% all the way down. Some people feel relief from snoring and puffiness right away, while others claim it takes six months to feel the full health benefits. And if 6 inches feels like too much, start with just an inch lift and work your way up.

Sleep Summary

The above practices can help you make the most of your sleep. Along with the benefits already described, studies also show that not getting enough quality sleep can increase your risk of obesity, high blood pressure, heart disease and even diabetes. It can weaken your immune system and deprive your body of restorative functions like muscle repair, protein and collagen synthesis and tissue repair in all areas of the body. Therefore, now I will recap some healthy sleep habits and add some extras, below.

✓The Solution:

Inclined Bed Therapy for healthy brain detoxification and circulation, healthy digestion and even fewer wrinkles.

Read books and leave your mobile phone outside of the room you sleep in. If you enjoy reading to help you relax, read from a real book so the adverse effects of the blue light will not interfere with your sleep.

Total darkness is key to sleeping well. That's because darkness signals the body that it's time to rest, while light suppresses the production of melatonin, the sleep-inducing hormone. At the same time, it turns out that the body requires darkness for optimal immune function, because melatonin doesn't just help you sleep, it plays a role in stopping cancer cells from growing.

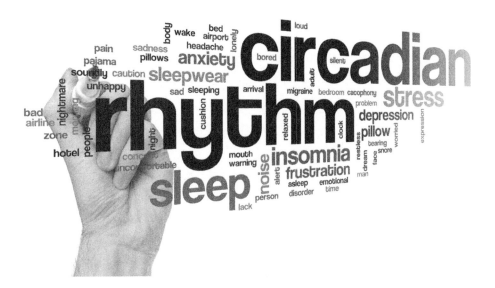

Make your sleeping time a habit. Studies show that those who go to bed at the same time each night are healthier. This may be because our bodies rely on circadian rhythms, with different functions being performed at specific times in accordance with the sun cycle. For example, there are times during the day when your digestive enzymes are more active, and nighttime is not one of them. When we create patterns in our lives, our bodies can better predict when to stimulate which function, and routine is key for healthy immunity, growth, healing and mental health.

Use Blue Blocking Glasses. Use good quality blue blocking glasses after sundown to eliminate the ill effects of blue light from your environment and electric devices, if you're using them.

Have a bedtime routine. Humans are creatures of habit, so when we create a healthy bedtime routine, it signals the hormones and other neurotransmitters that it will soon be time to fall asleep. Your bedtime routine can be anything you like. Some people read, some take a bath and others go for a walk, then read. If you enjoy television or movies, enjoy it, then turn off the TV and read for a while to allow your brain time to unwind. Also try to wake up at the same time each morning, even on weekends or on vacation. This helps your body stay on a 24-hour cycle, and you just might find more things to enjoy if you are out of town!

One of the reasons people get old—lose their aliveness—is that they get weighed down by all of their stuff.

—Richard Leider

CHAPTER 2

Ageless Hair & Teeth

How we see ourselves in the mirror has a tremendous impact on our outlook, feelings, confidence levels, and even our mood. How we feel can also show in our outward appearance. Unhappy or depressed people sometimes take their health (and looks) for granted. Some claim that appearance, whether it be fashion or personal, is frivolous. This simply isn't true.

Our appearance has a direct impact on how we feel. Looking our best can build self-confidence and even make us feel more energetic and attractive. Aside from appearance, neglecting personal health, including the health of our hair and teeth, can lead to long-term health problems; as how we look can indicate internal health issues.

Hair Health

Healthy, shiny hair is a sign of good health and a symbol of youth, and with just a few tweaks we can achieve incredible changes. At the same time, unhealthy hair may be a sign of nutritional deficiencies, underlying health issues or hormonal imbalances. Paying attention to our hair can help us stay healthy while giving us the confidence we wish to project.

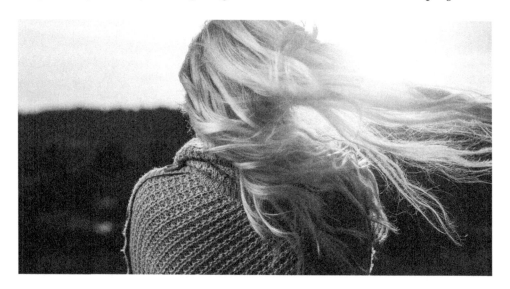

Frizzy Hair Can Age You

As we age, hair becomes dry and brittle, due to a lack of oils in the scalp, hormonal changes and hair that is less nourished. And face it, gray hair is a completely different texture than our "normal" color hair, and tends to be courser with less shine and curl. But that doesn't mean we have to live with it.

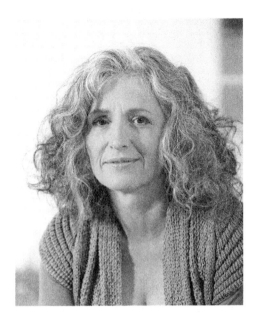

It may take a little effort, but there are healthy habits that you can do to help hair become more nourished and less frizzy. Here are some of them.

✓ The Solution

- **Support your thyroid.** The thyroid is responsible for the manufacturing of certain hormones that are associated with hair growth. When sluggish, your thyroid produces less of these, which can affect the quality of your hair. Talk to your doctor about getting your thyroid checked, or look for thyroid supporting supplements in your local health food store.

- **Keep your hair shorter.** Sometimes frizzy hair is simply the result of dry ends, or because as we age, the hair grows out thinner and shorter. Keeping your hair shorter and more manageable will keep it healthy looking.

- **Be sure you are consuming enough high-quality protein.** As we age, our bodies require more protein to keep up with the process of collagen production and tissue repair (even on the scalp).

Some women find that their hair loses volume and length after menopause. This is because menopause causes your estrogen levels to decrease. Estrogen is a hair-friendly hormone, helping to keep your hair in its growth phase for longer. You may also find that your hair breaks and becomes more frizzy and brittle after menopause.

- **Use an oil treatment once or twice a week.** This can be a hot oil treatment to condition your hair, or one that you massage in, like castor oil, Brahmi oil or coconut oil. Leave it in for a few hours or overnight and then wash and rinse. Check out my video for more info:

Channel: The Aging Games
Castor Oil for Hair Growth | Grow long Eyelashes and thick Eyebrows

- **Brush your hair while holding your head upside down** at least three times each week. This helps bring blood flow to the scalp, which brings more nutrients and oxygen to nutritionally deprived hair. *Bending over your bathtub will allow you to keep the hairs confined so they don't fly all over the bathroom.

- **Prevent Heat Damage.** Be careful with blow-drying and using straighteners and curling irons on a regular basis, as these will cause permanent damage to the hair structure.

- **Use Natural Hair Coloring Products.** Hair color can be very harsh and damaging to hair. Try to look for natural alternatives and color without the use of ammonia.

- **Try Platelet Rich Plasma (PRP).** PRP is derived from your blood and injected into your scalp. This treatment helps combat hair loss, increases hair growth, and completely changes the quality of your hair. Please see my video for more info:

Channel: The Aging Games
Stop Hair Loss with Platelet Rich Plasma PRP | Does it work?

Anti-Aging Haircuts

Adding soft layers to your hair can make you appear younger, while loose waves are younger-looking than straight hair. Soft layers will frame your face and give your hair natural bounce and volume. Of course, each person is different, so talk to your stylist, or try a new look, because there are many hairstyles that can seemingly remove years. Here are some of them.

✓ The Solution

- For some, a shorter haircut might just be that "non-surgical" facelift they were looking for. Hair that is chin-length or shorter can draw eyes away from facial drooping and perk up the face.

- Styling your hair away from your face can help you appear fresher.

- Bangs can be a cheap and safe alternative to Botox and can cover frown and forehead wrinkles. If you wear bangs, go for a wispy look or swoop them to the side. This way you still accentuate your eyes and cheekbones without hiding.

- If you keep your hair longer, don't forget to layer it for movement. Wearing it past the shoulders may be the best option for some to pre-

An increase in androgens in females can actually change the shape of the hair follicle from round to flat, and this can instigate a change in texture from straight to curly.

vent the "frizzy triangle" look. Keeping your hair longer with layers will add weight to the hair, preventing this look.

- If your hair tends to be limp or thin, try a shorter style with layers, swept to the side off your face. This can add volume, especially if you primp it while it's drying. Find the best part by separating your hair or bangs at the highest point of your eyebrow arch to bring out your eyes.

Hair Color

Darker colors can be quite aging for some, so after a certain age, experiment with a couple of shades lighter than your natural hair color. If you have a lot of gray, maintaining your roots can be particularly challenging with darker hair. A natural shade of blond or some blond highlights can really help mask those roots and give you more time between coloring treatments. As a general rule of thumb in the beauty world, lighter shades can make anyone look younger.

When choosing the right shade, avoid overly ashy tones. Instead, go for warmth with golden or auburn highlights. Talk to a color specialist to see what the best shade is for you. For example, honey tones can create a more youthful glow to one's complexion. If you prefer to work with your dark hair (or keep it dark), look for rich, chocolate colors that can add warmth to your skin.

You can also embrace and grow out your beautiful gray hair, which is a very popular trend nowadays. Use a toner to get rid of any brassiness and make sure you keep your lovely mane in tip top condition with regular treatments.

Dental Health

Some people never consider how the appearance and condition of our teeth can age us. But as we get older, teeth can become discolored due to years of coffee and wine consumption, stained from berries, or just yellowed with time. In addition, the health of our teeth can make a difference in our health. The following are some things to consider when it comes to keeping your mouth fresh, healthy, and youthful.

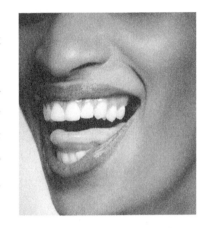

Mercury or Amalgam Fillings

If you have dental fillings, you may have a composite resin that looks like your natural teeth, or you may have the less pricey silver-looking fillings called amalgam (also referred to as mercury or silver fillings). This type of dental filling material is actually made of a combination of metals, which usually consists of a combination of mercury along with a mixture of silver, copper and/or tin. Even though it's been common knowledge for decades that they can seriously impact our health, they are still used by some dentists as a cost-effective way to fill cavities. After years of pressure from

Age is an issue of mind over matter. If you don't mind, it doesn't matter.

—**Mark Twain**

Consumers for Dental Choice and its allies, the FDA finally admits that dental amalgam releases mercury vapor that can cause health problems in some individuals.

Mercury fillings have been completely banned in Germany, Sweden, Norway and Denmark. At the same time, some groups like The International Academy of Oral Medicine and Toxicology (IAOMT), which includes scientists and dentists, believe there are numerous health risks associated with amalgam fillings. The claim that scientific studies show a correlation between mercury in fillings and the following health issues:

- Chronic Fatigue Syndrome (CFS)
- Autoimmune disorders
- Parkinson's disease
- Thyroiditis
- Kidney disease
- Periodontal disease
- Alzheimer's Disease

These are just a few on their list.[1] Each person has a unique sensitivity to mercury, and there are other factors that play a role in how your fillings will affect you, including the age of the filling, state of the filling (such as is it cracked) and health of the filled tooth and surrounding teeth. Sometimes the discoloration is so prominent that it can leech to the teeth near the one that is filled.

Sufficient sleep, exercise, healthy food, friendship, and peace of mind are necessities, not luxuries.

—**Mark Halperin**

Another issue with amalgam fillings is that they are supposed to be changed periodically, because they are prone to "fail" from the constant pressure of

---

1   Moore, R. (2020, October 16). Dental Amalgam Danger: Mercury Fillings and Human Health. Retrieved October 26, 2020, from **https://iaomt.org/resources/dental-mercury-facts/amalgam-fillings-danger-human-health/**

chewing, which can lead to the tooth cracking or breaking. Fillings can detach from the tooth, allowing bacteria to become trapped in between, leading to further decay and even tooth loss. Last, mercury fillings will eventually cause discoloration of the entire tooth, leaving it a bluish gray or blackish gray, in some cases.

And to make these fillings even more hazardous, as you drink and eat, especially warm food or liquids, the mercury gases release from the filling and are absorbed directly into the brain and other organs. This is why mercury fillings contribute to overall toxicity and various neurological issues.

According to Dr. Mercola, "Mercury has been mankind's preferred poison for decades. The phrase "mad as a hatter" originated from the radical personality changes "hatters" in the 1900s experienced the longer they worked with a mercury compound they applied on hats."

√The Solution

Luckily, today there are many dentists that will remove the fillings and replace them with the better looking and safer composite resin or porcelain, both of which are more natural looking. Be sure to find a good holistic dentist who takes precautions, such as ensuring the mercury or amalgam is not accidentally pushed into your system during removal. Ventilation and a well-placed dam inside your mouth are essential during the removal process. Once you have changed to healthier fillings, do a whole-body detox to help your body remove stored mercury. A whole-body detox can be performed through diet, supplements, homeopathic remedies and/or chelation therapy (either oral or IV).

The Color of Teeth

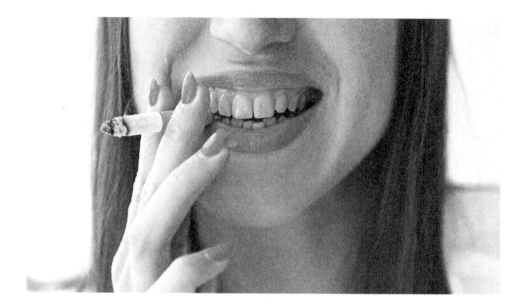

Aging is a process that affects the entire body, including teeth. As we age, we lose mineral in our teeth, while sugary and acidic foods can exacerbate the problem. Aging teeth can become stained due to certain food and drinks, while some medications can also cause discoloration. They can also become darkened as the enamel wears away, exposing the darker colored dentin underneath. Worse yet, teeth can become a gray color due to a combination of these. But there are many ways to treat this problem.

✓ The Solution

Of course, regular dental hygiene will slow the aging progression of the teeth. But there are other things that can help, too.

- Remineralize your teeth with special tooth powders and mouth washes for that purpose. These may include ingredients like charcoal, essential oils, bentonite clay, calcium carbonate, baking soda and sea salt. These products are used by many to help strengthen teeth and bring back their natural, healthy color.

- Regular Oil Pulling can also whiten and strengthen your teeth and improve overall dental health. Check out my video for more info:

Channel: The Aging Games
Oil Pulling for Whiter Teeth and Improved Health

- Talk to your dentist about tooth whitening. A dentist can oversee the process and ensure you get the right amount of whitening for your complexion and teeth. There are dentists today that are more holistic and can help guide you to non-toxic tooth whitening products with ingredients that don't harm you or your teeth. Be very cautious with this process as continued bleaching can harm your enamel and actually make teeth look much worse over the years. Be especially careful with home bleaching kits.

Worn Down Teeth with Age and Grinding

Due to grinding, clenching, or just overuse, our teeth eventually become shorter, stubbier and our bite and jaw alignment can change dramatically. This can eventually lead to an overbite, problems with chewing, and also bring on premature aging to the lower face. It can cause the jaw to recede and for jowls and sagging to form.

One famous dentist in California, Dr. Muslin, has pioneered a procedure

I suppose real old age begins when one looks backward rather than forward.

—**Mary Sarton**

When your teeth are badly worn down, they don't always fit together properly. This misalignment can cause severe strain in your jaw, and this strain can radiate and lead to headaches, TMJ and even Trigeminal Neuralgia.

called Facelift Dentistry, where he restores teeth to their original size and fixes many types of bite issues as well as aesthetic issues with dental tabletops and veneers. By improving the way the teeth look and function, he's able to make patients look 10 or even 20 years younger.

Stop Using Fluoride

Ceasing the use of fluoride products for dental hygiene might sound counterintuitive for many people, as we have been brainwashed to include fluoride every chance we get. It is an ingredient in most toothpastes and mouthwashes and some dentists will provide extra fluoride pills for those whom they feel need it. In addition to our "normal" intake of fluoride, states in many countries have taken it upon themselves to add it to our drinking water "for our own good."

Unfortunately, over 400 studies have demonstrated that fluoride is a neurotoxin and has no place in the human body. Fluoride's ability to damage the brain is one of the most active areas of fluoride research today. In fact, it accumulates and builds up in the body.

The fluoride in drinking water, as it is actually fluorosilicic acid (FSA), a liquid waste and inorganic fluoride compound that may also contain lead and arsenic.[2] This type of fluoride is a toxin that affects the nervous system, and is associated with thyroid problems, osteoarthritis, gastrointestinal problems and reproductive issue in younger people.

While some groups like the Centers for Disease Control claim there is no evidence that links fluoride to health problems, other groups like Fluoride Alert claim there are numerous health issues linked to excess fluoride in the body, especially FSA. One problem they point out is that according to the U.S. Department of Health and Human Services, too much fluoride can result in skeletal fluorosis, a bone disease which is often diagnosed as arthritis or chronic joint pain. A large-scale study in China found that incidents of osteoarthritis increased with fluoride levels in the body.[3]

Of all the self-fulfilling prophecies in our culture the assumption that aging means decline and poor health is probably the deadliest.

—Marilyn Ferguson

✓ The Solution

- Fluoride is used to remineralize teeth, however there are safer ways to do so, such as the tooth powders and rinses mentioned above. Simply search online or at your local health food market for "tooth remineralization" products.

- Research the drinking water in your area to determine the source of fluoride and amount. This can help you determine if you should switch to another drinking water that contains only natural fluoride.

---

2   Toxic Treatment: The Story of Fluoride. (2020, January). Retrieved October 26, 2020, from http://origins.osu.edu/article/toxic-treatment-fluorides-transformation-industrial-waste-public-health-miracle

3   Health Effects. (2019, September 14). Retrieved October 26, 2020, from http://fluoridealert.org/issues/health/

Fluoride seems to fit in with lead, mercury, and other poisons that cause chemical brain drain. All of these toxic chemicals will lead to premature aging of the body.

(Keep in mind if you do see a fluoride level in water that has none added, it is a natural, and thus more bio-available type.)

- Avoid cooking with non-stick cookware as these products can increase fluoride intake.

- Avoid fluoride treatments from the dentist.

- Reduce tea consumption or drink tea with younger leaves (they absorb less fluoride from watering).

- Drink only organic grape juice and wine.

- Consume less processed foods on a daily basis; opt for fresh, whole foods.

Oil Pulling for Healthy Teeth and Gums

Oil pulling is a practice that has been used for thousands of years, and often promoted by those who practice Ayurveda, an ancient healing art in India. Harmful microorganisms that can cause decay and infection are covered with a fatty membrane of the cell's skin, which cause decay and infection. But when these pathogens come into contact with the oil, they adhere to it until the oil is rinsed from the mouth.

The reported benefits of oil pulling include whiter teeth, prevention of cavities, and stronger teeth and gums. Some also believe it can help alleviate sinus infections and other problems with the nose and sinuses as the oil helps attract and remove trapped bacteria.

✓The Solution

While different oils may be used, it's best to avoid those that contain too much omega-6, which can be pro inflammatory. The best option is organic coconut oil, as it contains vitamins A, D, E and K. It also contains the lauric acid, which is often used to treat both bacterial and viral infections.

To do oil pulling, take about 1 Tablespoon of coconut oil into your mouth and gently swish it around for 20 minutes. Some people might prefer to begin with 1 teaspoon and work their way up and even try 5 minutes and work up to 20. When you are done, spit the oil into a trash receptacle so it doesn't harden and clog your sink. More info on oil pulling here:

Channel: The Aging Games
Castor Oil for Hair Growth | Grow long Eyelashes and thick Eyebrows

Conclusion

Of course, seeing your dentist and hairdresser regularly and consuming a healthy diet free of sugars and other highly processed foods will also support the health of your teeth and hair. If you need to adjust your diet over time, incorporating some of these tips and hacks can help you keep your teeth and hair youthful and beautiful.

CHAPTER 3

How to Create an Anti-Aging Diet

Diet is one of the most important ways to slow the aging process, ward off disease, keep up energy levels and to simply feel great. Our diet is the basis of health and the nutrients from our diet are what the body uses to make new, fresh cells for all parts of our body, including healthy skin and healthy organs.

On the other hand, harmful foods like those that are full of sugar or are highly processed can accelerate the aging process, compromise your immune system, and make your skin look older than your years. An old saying that fitness trainers often tell their clients is that "abs are made in the kitchen". That's because the healthy building blocks of nutrition are used to help the body repair and build muscle, while helping the liver burn fat for optimal health.

Age is no barrier. It's a limitation you put on your mind.

—Jackie Joyner-Kersee

As we get older, our digestion slows down and may not work as well as when we were younger. During the menopausal years, hormones get out of whack, interfering with sleep, energy and weight loss efforts. This makes it even more important to consume the right foods that help our bodies keep up daily maintenance and repair.

Keep in mind that our immune system needs more help as we age, while collagen production and protein synthesis also slow down. Nutrition is the cornerstone of support for these processes, allowing them to continue to run efficiently. The following tips are not about what foods are anti-aging, but instead are nutritional guidelines to support all of your body's functions. These guidelines will help you make conscious choices for your individual, daily nutritional needs.

Natural Diabetes Prevention and Weight Control

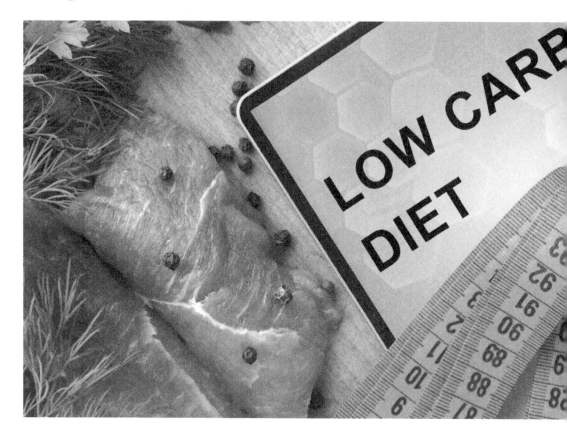

It is possible to lower your insulin and blood sugar levels naturally through diet. Insulin is a hormone that helps keep blood sugar levels in check, and in an ideal world there should be balance between insulin and blood sugar. Too little insulin will cause blood sugar levels that are too high, which can damage parts of the body, mainly the kidneys.

On the other hand, too much insulin is linked to obesity, heart disease, and cancer. Insulin resistance is a common condition for many people today, and is a result of consistently too much insulin in the body. High insulin makes the body resistant to the effects of the hormone, so your body produces even more in an attempt to stimulate an effect. This cycle is where people run into the most health problems. But there are ways to naturally reduce insulin levels, which can also help you maintain a healthy weight at any age.

✔ The Solution

Follow a low-carb diet, because many studies confirm these types of diets are not only effective for weight loss, but help lower insulin levels in the blood and increase your sensitivity to insulin. This is because carbohydrates raise blood sugar more than proteins and fats, and long-term consumption of refined carbohydrates will put one in a state of insulin resistance. But resistance isn't futile.

Your 40s are good. Your 50s are great. Your 60s are fab. And 70 is f*@king awesome!

—Helen Mirren

In order to lose weight and prevent diabetes, your carbs should be under 20 grams per day. There are different schools of thought when it comes to fat and protein. Some experts swear by a high fat diet, which would involve 70% or more of your daily intake of calories coming from fat. Some people do great with this ratio and lose weight very rapidly, while others have to decrease their fat a bit lower to achieve the same results.

The same thing is true for protein. Some women do great with high protein, moderate fat and low carb. Others do better with moderate protein, high fat, and low carbs. The common denominator is "low carbs," so I'd suggest sorting this out first and then playing with your protein and

According to WebMD: Research suggests that people with type 2 diabetes can slim down and lower their blood sugar levels with the keto diet. In one study, people with type 2 lost weight, needed less medication, and lowered their A1c when they followed the keto diet for a year.

fat intake until you find your sweet spot. This is the place where you feel great, full of energy, and you are losing weight or maintaining if that's your goal.

Low Carb/Keto/Paleo diets are all associated with helping post-menopausal women improve (lower) their blood glucose levels and are now recommended for anyone who desires to lower insulin. But there are still other practices you can do.

- Consume small amounts of apple cider vinegar each day by adding 1-2 teaspoons on a salad or other dish. In fact, 2 teaspoons after a high-carb meal can lower insulin levels, but I would not recommend using this in lieu of cutting down on your refined carbs.

- Don't snack, instead fast between meals, the longer these fasts are the better. See Intermittent Fasting for more info also check out my video:

Channel: The Aging Games
Intermittent Fasting | 5 Common Mistakes that Prevent Weight Loss

- Avoid sugar in any form, including most fruits (more on this later)

- Exercise three to five times each week, focusing on weight training, stretching, walking, etc.

- Use cinnamon in cooking or take a cinnamon supplements (again, while this can help you enjoy a treat once in a while, it is not a replacement for lowering carb intake)

Cholesterol is Your Friend

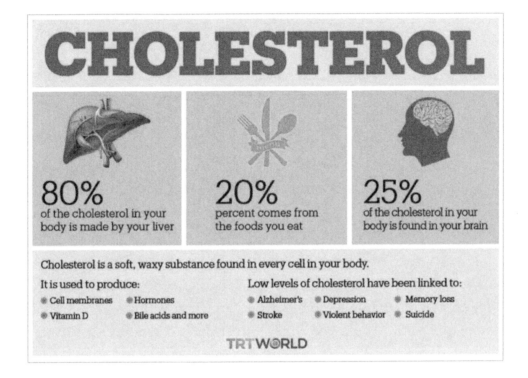

Don't fear cholesterol because it turns out that women and men with higher cholesterol live longer. We have traditionally been told that there are two forms of cholesterol: one is good (HDL) and the other is bad (LDL) or harmful to our health. It turns out that this may be wrong.

An international team of experts reviewed a series of studies, which involved over 68,000 participants over 60 years of age. Surprisingly, the studies found that elderly people with higher LDL lived longer than those with lower. Another study by researchers at the Norwegian University of Science and Technology found that women with high cholesterol (greater than 270 mg/dl) had a 28% lower mortality rate than those with lower cholesterol of less than 183 mg/dl.[1][2]

Most of the cholesterol in your body, in fact 80%, is made by your liver, while only 20% comes from food. Now think about this for a moment. Would your liver be producing something that is going to kill you? Of course not! Our brain is made of cholesterol, our bodies need cholesterol to produce hormones and for various bodily functions. According to The Weston A. Price Foundation, fat and cholesterol are very important components in human milk. In fact, the milk from a healthy mother has about 50 to 60 percent of its energy as fat.

Know that you are the perfect age. Each year is special and precious, for you shall only live it once. Be comfortable with growing older.

—Louise Hay

The cholesterol in human milk supplies an infant with close to six times the amount most adults consume from their food today. Does it make any sense that as babies, cholesterol is essential to our development and then it would be harmful for the remaining of our lives? Making people believe that cholesterol is harmful is one of the biggest cons in medicine of the 20th century.

1   University of South Florida (USF Innovation). (2016, June 27). No association between 'bad cholesterol' and elderly deaths: Systematic review of studies of over 68,000 elderly people also raises questions about the benefits of statin drug treatments. ScienceDaily. Retrieved October 26, 2020 from www.sciencedaily.com/releases/2016/06/160627095006.htm

2   Petursson H, Sigurdsson JA, Bengtsson C, Nilsen TI, Getz L. Is the use of cholesterol in mortality risk algorithms in clinical guidelines valid? Ten years prospective data from the Norwegian HUNT 2 study. J Eval Clin Pract. 2012 Feb;18(1):159-68. doi: 10.1111/j.1365-2753.2011.01767.x. Epub 2011 Sep 25. PMID: 21951982; PMCID: PMC3303886.

I know what you're thinking! But what about cholesterol blocking my arteries? What about my heart? If you want to know why cholesterol is found in the arteries, it's not because it's trying to block them, it's actually there to repair the damage caused by processed carbs, sugar and toxic vegetable oils and margarine. Inflammation damages arterial walls and contributes to cardiovascular problems. Cholesterol is the repair molecule that comes in and tries to fix the damage. A bigger concern should be chronic, internal inflammation, not high cholesterol.

This does not mean we can go out and eat as much fatty foods and junk foods as we like and expect to live longer. Fats should always come from a healthy source, and saturated fats (from animal sources or coconut oil) are actually good for your health.

The most important anti-aging diet strategy should be to stop eating fast food. Check the ingredients list for "partially hydrogenated" or "hydrogenated" oils on all packaged foods from the supermarket. If either of these dangerous oils are listed, don't eat it. Look in particular at margarines, cookies, cakes, pastries, doughnuts, and fast food. And as I mention throughout this book (see chapter 4), "Sugar is a far worse threat to your heart than fat ever was."

"CRP is a marker for inflammation that is directly associated with overall heart and cardiovascular health. In multiple studies, CRP has been identified as a potent predictor of future cardiovascular health"

— Jonny Bowden, *The Great Cholesterol Myth: Why Lowering Your Cholesterol Won't Prevent Heart Disease-and the Statin-Free Plan That Will*

✔ The Solution

Decrease inflammation in your body!

Pay more attention to the types of foods you eat, always aiming for wholesome, high quality foods. This means foods that are not processed and packed with nutrition.

For example, don't be afraid of healthy fats from avocados and olive oil, but do worry about the fats in fast food French fries and processed pastries. If you're a vegan, choose healthy protein alternatives to meat like pea proteins, sprouts, nuts and seeds over processed "veggie burgers" that contain the highly toxic TVP, or textured vegetable protein, which is a junk food.

Oh, the worst of all tragedies is not to die young, but to live until I am seventy-five and yet not ever truly to have lived.

—Martin Luther King Jr.

Eat More Fat

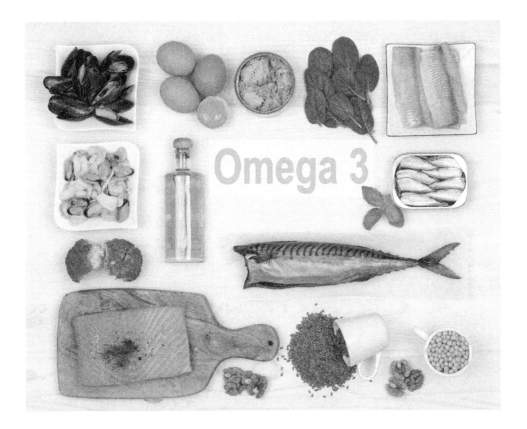

Healthy fats have many health benefits, especially for the mature body. Consuming healthy fats can literally preserve our brain and other organs, and help slow the aging process. They can help lower our risk for heart disease, prevent abnormal heart rhythm, lower blood pressure and improve our mood and outlook on life. But, as mentioned above, choose quality fats over unhealthy ones. Here I will describe the difference.

Fats are necessary for good health. They play a role in brain function, lubricating the body, and help break down fat-soluble vitamins. They can add a healthy sheen to skin and give hair an added gloss. And not having enough of the right fats can cause health issues like depression and hormonal issues.

Fats are divided into groups including saturated and unsaturated fats, trans fats and Omega-3, Omega 6 and Omega 9. And to make matters more confusing, we have monounsaturated and polyunsaturated. Here is a breakdown of each:

Saturated fats have wrongly been viewed as the villains of fats, mainly due to the misconception about cholesterol and heart disease. It all began with the flawed but infamous Seven Countries Study in the mid-1900s. The study included Finland, Greece, US, Italy, Yugoslavia, Netherlands and Japan investigating links between coronary heart disease mortality and lifestyle factors, especially the intake of saturated fatty acids. The "diet-heart hypothesis" demonstrated that vegetable oils lowered total blood cholesterol levels by an average of 14 percent.

The problem was that this lowered cholesterol did not actually help people live longer. Instead, the lower cholesterol fell, the higher the risk of dying: 22 percent higher for every 30-point fall. Participants also failed to demonstrate having less atherosclerosis or fewer heart attacks. Another flaw in this research was the fact that they actually began with 22 countries, but the ones that didn't fit the hypothesis were disregarded, reducing the study to only 7 countries.

You don't stop laughing when you grow old, you grow old when you stop laughing.

—George Bernard Shaw

With a political agenda and millions of dollars donated to the American Heart Association (AHA) (by the food industry producing vegetable oils and low-fat grain-based foods), the Seven Countries Study was hugely influential in new guidelines advising against eating saturated fat and arguing for the benefits of polyunsaturated fats.

Fast forward to 2020 and according to Dr. Paul Saladino, MD, saturated fat, especially long chain saturated fats, like those found in red meat from ruminants, are the most healthy fats you can eat while chicken and pork fed corn can actually harm you. What happens when animals are fed corn? The meat becomes high in omega-6 linoleic acid, as corn is high in this type of fat. Please check out this podcast from Dr. Saladino for more info: **https://bengreenfieldfitness.com/transcripts/transcript-the-carnivore-diet/**

Unsaturated fats were generally thought to be healthy and necessary for good health. These include both monounsaturated and polyunsaturated fats, and may be found in seeds, vegetable oils, nuts, and some fish like salmon. Omega 3 is a polyunsaturated fat found in foods such as fish, walnuts, and flaxseeds.

So let's talk about vegetable oils for a moment. Corn, canola, soy, and peanut oils are commonly used by people for cooking, thinking they're heart-healthy alternatives to animal fats. What they don't realize is that all of these oils are actually highly inflammatory. Please check out this link to find out more about the health implications of using vegetable oils: **https://carnivoreaurelius.com/why-is-vegetable-oil-bad-for-you/**

Other than vegetable oils, the main source of polyunsaturated fats are almonds, nuts, and seeds, all of which are high in an Omega-6 fatty acid called linoleic acid. Excessive intake of linoleic acid in the diet can serve as a signal for humans to start storing fat for the winter. According to Dr. Saladino, linoleic acid is an evolutionary signal to our brains that winter is coming, and you better get fat and insulin-resistant, so you can survive a lean winter, except winter never comes for us because we always have food at the grocery store in the same amount.

Trans fats are the worst for your health. They are liquid at room temperatures, so food manufacturers add hydrogen to make them more appealing (spreadable), which turns it into a hydrogenated fat. This unnatural chemical alteration leads to increased internal inflammation, leaving you at risk for a host of diseases, and is a major contributor to heart disease. Some of these foods include margarine, fried foods, ready-to-use dough, vegetable shortening, coffee creamers and most baked goods. According to Dr. Saladino, "increasingly, we're finding that trans fats and polyunsaturated fat from vegetable oils are far worse for your health, and a greater contributor to chronic disease, than added sugar even."

Omega 3's are polyunsaturated fats, as mentioned above. There are three major ones called EPA, DHA and ALA. These fats improve heart health, mental health, weight control, and can even help decrease fatty livers. These are necessary for optimal health and the best source is from eggs, seafood and cold-water fatty fish, such as salmon, mackerel, herring, and sardines. Be careful with Omega 3 supplements as fish oil in capsules can quickly become rancid and cause all kinds of health issues.

Omega 6's fatty acids are also polyunsaturated fats and essential to good health, with the most prevalent Omega 6 being linoleic acid. But remember Dr. Saladino's warning about excess linoleic acid? These types of fats are found in walnuts, hemp seeds, sunflower seeds, peanut butter and avocadoes. But they are also found in fast food, cured meats and processed snacks. While the fat itself is necessary for good health, it is now believed that a proper balance is required of a 1:1 ratio from Omega 6 and Omega 3. Hunter gatherers ate an approximately 1:1 ratio. Because of seed oils, the Standard American Diet is closer to 20:1. This sets you up for disease, discomfort and premature aging.

✓The Solution

With so many fats to pay attention to, how do we keep track? We have been taught to fear animal fats and praise the fats in nuts, seeds, grains, legumes and soy. The fact is that these foods are cheap to produce and do not actually support human health.

Depending on the type of diet you're doing, your fat intake will vary. Calculating macronutrients and calories is not an easy task, but also not necessary in my opinion. I'm a big fan of eating animal foods from nose to tail, thus including lots of healthy fats and organ meat. Fish and seafood should also be included in a healthy diet, thus providing a larger variety of healthy fats. In addition to this, you might want to add avocadoes, coconut oil, extra virgin olive oil, as well as butter and ghee.

> *Avocados are about 77% fat, making them even higher in fat than most animal foods.*

reduces fat in liver   prevents heart diseases   improves mental disorder

fights depression and anxiety   Omega 3 ?   improves sleep

improves bone and joint health   alleviates menstrual plan   improves eye health

Increase Protein Intake

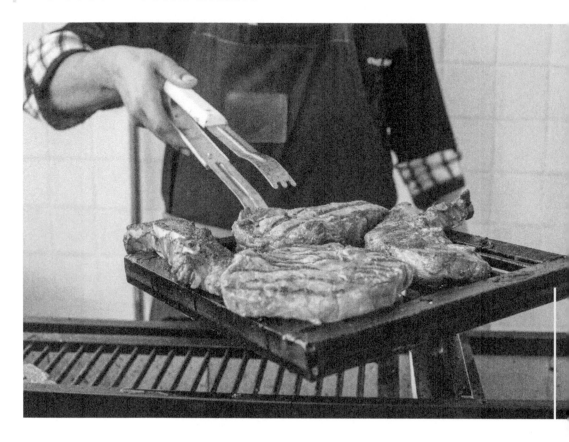

Recent research has revealed that as we age, our protein requirements increase. But this all-important macronutrient is so important to repair and build tissue throughout the body, including muscle and organ tissue. It is a necessary component of our bones, skin, muscles, hair, blood and cartilage. It is critical to help carry oxygen throughout the body, which gives us more energy. And it helps your body create antibodies that fight infection and ward off illness. This means we need it in just about every function our bodies undergo every day.

When we get older, our protein needs increase, especially with illness, during hospitalization and to prevent unwanted weight loss and sarcopenia (muscle deterioration). We also require more protein for strength and to preserve muscle mass. Even if you are healthy, chances are you require up to one-third more protein than when you were younger.

Unfortunately, many people consume less protein as digestion slows and they simply feel less hungry. Many other factors play a role in decreased protein intake, including dental issues, impaired taste or swallowing problems. When muscles deteriorate, it could create an unhealthy cycle of lessened appetite, so less protein is consumed, leading to further muscle deterioration and lowered appetite. At least one study found that those who have difficulty climbing stairs and walking were those who ate the least amount of protein. [3]

√ The Solution

Make protein, with a healthy portion of fat (think ribeye steak) the staple of your diet.

Here are some healthy sources of protein to fit into your daily regimen:

- High quality animal protein (grass fed, organic, etc.)

- Free range eggs

- Fatty fish and other seafood

- Drink bone broth on a regular basis

- Cheese and dairy products if you can tolerate them

---

3   Mendonça, N., Granic, A., Hill, T.R., Siervo, M., Mathers, J.C., Kingston, A. and Jagger, C. (2019), Protein Intake and Disability Trajectories in Very Old Adults: The Newcastle 85+ Study. J Am Geriatr Soc, 67: 50-56. doi:10.1111/jgs.15592

Whole eggs are actually loaded with vitamins and minerals. They contain a little bit of almost every single nutrient we need. They even contain powerful antioxidants that protect the eyes, and lots of choline, a brain nutrient that 90% of people don't get enough of.

Treat Fruit as a Treat

Treat fruit like the tasty dessert that it is, so consume it in moderation, only eat fruits that are in season and preferably organic. If you truly love fruit, keep it to no more than 1-2 servings a day, and aim for those with low sugar like berries, especially if you're watching your weight.

The health benefits of fruits come when the fruit is eaten whole, not ground up into a juice or smoothie. In fact, fruit juices and smoothies can stimulate the sweet tooth, because one smoothie can easily contain 18 grams or more of sugar.

While the sugar in fruit is natural, it is a form called fructose, which, when eaten in high amounts, may overwhelm the liver as it turns the fructose into fat. Some theories by naturalists believe that fruit contains fructose instead of glucose to trick animals into eating more as a way to spread the seeds!

Also keep in mind that most of the fruit we consume today does not and has never existed in nature. They've been genetically modified to be sweeter and prettier and more appealing to our eyes and taste buds.

Excessive fruit consumption can lead to:

• Weight Gain

• Fatty Liver

• Diabetes

• Digestive Issues (such as gas and bloating)

5 COMMON FOODS BEFORE AND AFTER HUMANS DOMESTICATED THEM

Wild watermelon
Judging by paintings of the fruit dating to the 17th century, watermelons may have once had seeds arranged in **swirly geometric patterns.**

Modern watermelon
Over time, humans have bred watermelons to have a **bright red**, juicy interior. The **seeds are often removed** by preventing the plants from being fertilized by pollination.

Wild banana
The first bananas may have been cultivated at least **7,000 years ago** in what is now Papua New Guinea, and were **stocky and hard**, with large, tough **seeds** throughout the fruit's interior.

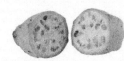

Modern banana
Today's tastier bananas are **hybrids** of two wild banana varieties, **Musa acuminata** and **Musa balbisiana.**

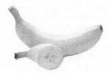

Wild eggplant
Eggplants once came in a wide array of shapes and colors, from **blue to yellow**, and some were **round** rather than oblong. Primitive eggplant varieties had a **spine** where the modern plant's stem connects to its flowers.

Modern eggplant
Selective breeding has made the **spine disappear** and left us with the **oblong purple** vegetable we're familiar with.

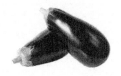

Wild carrot
The first carrots were likely cultivated around the 10th century in Asia Minor and were either **white or purple** with thin, forked roots and a **strong flavor.**

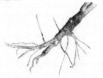

Modern carrot
Carrots today are large, **bright orange,** and tasty.

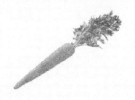

Wild corn
One of the most standout examples of selective breeding is North American sweet corn, which was bred from the barely edible **teosinte plant**. Natural corn was first domesticated around 7,000 BC and was thought to have been as **dry as a raw potato.**

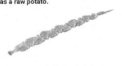

Modern corn
The corn we eat now is **1,000 times bigger** and much easier to grow and peel. A majority of these changes started taking shape after the 15th century, when **European settlers** started farming it.

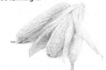

SOURCES: Dan L. Perlman/EcoLibrary; "History and Iconography of Eggplant," Chronica Horticulturae; "Tracing antiquity of banana cultivation in Papua New Guinea," The Australia & Pacific Science Foundation; Vox; World Carrot Museum

INSIDER

According to PubMed: Fructose has also been implicated as the main cause of symptoms in some patients with chronic diarrhea or other functional bowel disturbances. In addition, excessive fructose consumption may be responsible in part for the increasing prevalence of obesity, diabetes mellitus, and non-alcoholic fatty liver disease.

Vegetables

I know that this is a very sensitive topic and I don't want the reader to discredit everything else I've written in this book because you might disagree with me. I've followed the Keto, Paleo and other low-carb diets for most of my adult life, focusing on lots of vegetables. I was even vegetarian for 4 years. I really have done it all. However, the truth is that until I eliminated most veggies from my diet; I wasn't able to heal and lose weight. Through the groups I'm in, I've been able to interact with thousands of people who are in a similar boat.

If you love your veggies and they agree with you, you feel healthy and happy and at your ideal weight, then please just skip over to the next topic. If not, then please keep an open mind.

Anyone who keeps the ability to see beauty never grows old.

—Franz Kafka

Humans are able to survive off of animal products alone. We cannot say the same about plants or carbohydrates. (Even though some vegans are doing this, they need to supplement with some essential nutrients, such as B12, which is only found in animal foods.) As with fruit above, most of the vegetables we eat today do not exist in nature, and therefore our ancestors did not consume them. Also, unlike animals, plants are not able to run away from their prey so they need to produce certain substances to keep predators away.

According to The European Prospective Investigation into Cancer study, which ran for over 30 years studying the possibility that fruit and vegetables may help reduce the risk of cancer, but no protective effects have been firmly established.

So where exactly did we get the idea that we need to be eating 5 servings of fruit and vegetables each day? It actually originated back in 1991 in California during a meeting of the Produce for Better Health Foundation, American National Cancer Institute (ANCI), and 25 major fruit and vegetable companies. There were no nutritionists or scientists present, and the agenda was purely based on how to get more produce to the consumer. It wasn't actually about improving the health of the population.

The trouble is, when a number—your age—becomes your identity, you've given away your power to choose your future.

—Richard J. Leider

But the best argument I have against eating vegetables is the fact that it's the first food that we try to feed babies and all babies absolutely despise it. Unless veggies are hidden under a mountain of cheese, cream or dressing, they're actually not very palatable. Now show me one other animal that doesn't naturally gravitate to and enjoy its natural food. Show me a cow that turns its nose up at the sight of grass or a lion that prefers bananas over meat. So why do we need to grow up before we can actually enjoy some vegetables (usually smothered in butter) and why do we only have one stomach to digest them?

Some common toxins found in vegetables that can be detrimental to human health are phytic acid, oxalates, lectins and glycoalkaloids. This mixture of chemicals, proteins, and acids can not only damage our sensitive digestive system but can also lead to hormonal imbalances and contribute to different autoimmune conditions. [4]

4   Schoenfeld, B.J., Aragon, A.A. How much protein can the body use in a single meal for muscle-building? Implications for daily protein distribution. J Int Soc Sports Nutr 15, 10 (2018). https://doi.org/10.1186/s12970-018-0215-1

Soy contains high levels of goitrogens. Goitrogens are compounds that inhibit the thyroid's ability to utilize iodine correctly, which could lead to hypothyroidism, causing your whole metabolism to slow down.

You might also be surprised to learn that most of the pesticides you consume do not actually come from the chemicals sprayed on your food, but from the chemicals the plant produces to ward off insects.

So based on this, do I never eat any vegetables? I actually didn't for a long time until I got my Hashimoto's and eczema under control and lost the weight I needed to lose. My diet is still based mostly on meat, fat and dairy but I do use the occasional veggie, mostly in flavoring while cooking or as a small side dish/garnish. This plan works for me and for many people that I know. It may not be for everyone though so as with everything, I encourage you to do your own research and to find the right meal plan for you.

My friend Carnivore Aurelius has a great summary about vegetables: https://carnivoreaurelius.com/vegetables/

Please check out this video about the Risks and Benefits of Eating Plants:

Channel: AncestryFoundation
AHS12 Georgia Ede MD Little Shop of Horrors? The Risks and Benefits of Eating Plants

Watch What You Drink

The beverages we drink can make or break a diet. Sadly, fruit juices, soft drinks, flavored coffees, smoothies and energy drinks, are not just empty calories but also very unhealthy. Replacing these with herbal teas and mineral water can have a very positive impact on your weight, state of mind and the aging process in general.

A Frappuccino can have 500 calories and 70 grams (6 tbsp) of sugar in a 16-ounce serving.

Check out my video about vitamin waters:

Channel: The Aging Games
Is Vitamin Water Healthy For You?

Alcohol Consumption

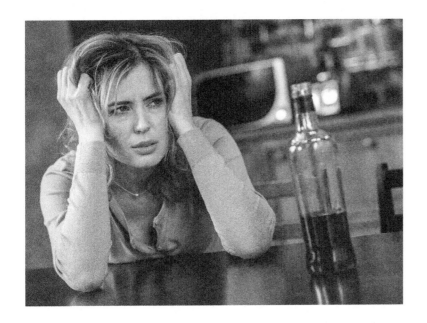

From an early age, all we see is alcohol everywhere. Just watch any movie or TV show and the actors are rarely standing or sitting around with an empty hand. There's usually a glass or red wine or some Whisky on the rocks to keep them pacified. Celebrations automatically include some form of alcohol, and we are conditioned to believe that drinking is the only way to unwind after a stressful day. It is much more culturally accepted and expected that we drink on a regular basis, than ever before. Those who don't take part in this ritual are often shunned or ridiculed and not invited out as they're "no fun."

I've always said that I will never let an old person into my body. That is, I don't believe in 'thinking' old. Don't program yourself to break down as you age with thoughts that decline is inevitable.

—**Wayne Dyer**

However, when it comes to aging gracefully, reducing your alcohol intake can ensure a longer, healthier life, more vibrant skin, well-shaped muscles and increased energy. And while many people drink to feel happier, alcohol is a depressant that can increase anxiety, stress and depressed episodes. Adverse physical effects also come with regular alcohol consumption. Some of these include increased risk for heart disease, irregular heartbeat, high blood pressure, cancer and liver disease, and it can cause your body to pack on fat as your liver becomes sluggish in an attempt to detoxify the alcohol. Since alcohol is viewed as a poison by the body, any time you drink alcohol, the liver shuts down the fat burning process for up to 48 hours in order to eliminate this toxin. So if you're watching your weight or trying to shed pounds but have reached a plateau, alcohol might very well be the culprit.

One incredible finding was that drinking more than 100 grams of alcohol a week was associated with a lowered life expectancy, and it is considered a level-one carcinogen (meaning there is strong evidence it can lead to cancer).

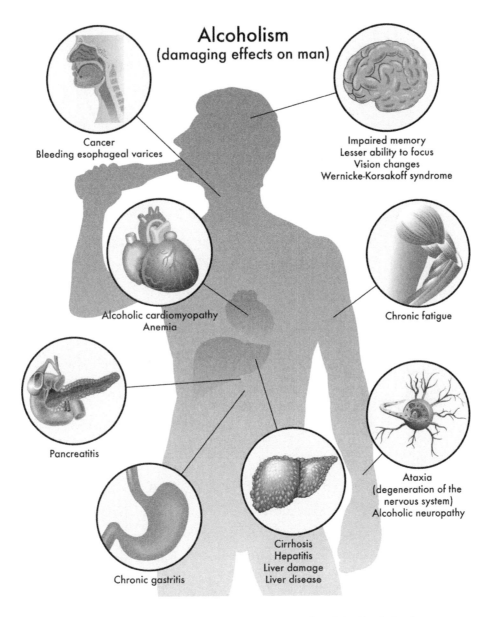

As we age, alcohol takes a bigger toll on our health. It dehydrates your entire body, leaving the skin less plump and tired looking. You know what

I'm talking about. Just as with smokers, you can always tell by looking at someone's face if they are drinkers. Even if you drink water to counteract the alcohol, it will not undo the damage that took place while drinking. Worse yet, alcohol has a direct impact on our vital organs and causes them to age quicker, which can put you in last place in The Aging Games.

> "
> It annoys me when people say, 'Even if you're old, you can be young at heart!' Hiding inside this well-meaning phrase is a deep cultural assumption that old is bad and young is good. What's wrong with being old at heart, I'd like to know? Wouldn't you like to be loved by people whose hearts have practiced loving for a long time?
>
> **—Susan Moon**

Some adults increase alcohol intake as they get older and close to retirement or as they enter retirement. This may feel like fun at first, but don't forget you have an exciting part of your life coming up. It can be easy to fall into the habit of drinking an entire bottle of wine every day, yet this can lead to sleeping difficulties and other issues.

Despite making your drowsy, alcohol is not a good sleep aid. In fact, it has a very negative effect on sleep patterns. Alcohol is a central nervous system depressant that slows down brain activity. It has a sedative effect on the system that can induce feelings of relaxation and sleepiness, but the consumption of alcohol has been linked to poor sleep quality and duration. With regular alcohol use, you'll be missing out on the important restorative REM sleep, which will lead to drowsiness and low concentration during the day.

Giving up alcohol altogether has been life changing for many people. They find new energy they never realized they had, health problems seem to dissipate and their overall outlook on life improves. Some begin exercising, while others take up hobbies. But the choice of how one reduces their alcohol intake is a very personal choice, and it does not affect everyone the same. At the same time, if alcohol interferes with your personal relationships, work or physical health, that may be a good indication to cut back or quit.

✓The Solution

Limit your alcohol intake to special occasions or stop drinking altogether. You will add years to your life, your skin will be smoother and more vibrant and you'll improve your sleep and cognitive function while reducing your chances or developing just about every major disease. Here are some other tips to follow:

- Keep a journal of your diet, including food and beverages. This will bring more awareness to your alcohol habits, as well as any other food habits that should be reconsidered.

- Skip socializing at the bar and join a class or gym instead. If your regular routine involves having drinks with your significant other during dinner, schedule a walk or gym session to help motivate you to not drink alcohol.

- Practice drinking only in certain social situations and stick with it.

Chronic consumption of alcohol disrupts the communication between nervous, endocrine and immune system and causes hormonal disturbances that lead to serious consequences at physiological and behavioral levels.

Those who love deeply never grow old; they may die of old age, but they die young.

—Ben Franklin

- Avoid the after-work drinks with coworkers and engage in other social activities instead.

- Never drink if you feel sad or depressed, as alcohol can intensify these feelings.

- When you do go out for cocktails with friends, keep a glass of water on hand to sip from, because sipping the drink can become a nervous habit or you might just be thirsty!

- Back to the journaling. If you decide to abstain from alcohol altogether to experiment with a dry month, keep track of how you feel each day and notice the benefits.

Water

Water is the essence of life. We use it to hydrate, cook, bathe, shower and brush our teeth. Consuming enough water helps deliver nutrients throughout the body, including the skin. Because of this, it plays a role in helping skin replenish itself and maintain elasticity or firmness, which can help delay signs of aging like wrinkles. But we have a problem with today's water. Tap water is not as clean or healthy as some might believe, but bottled water has issues, too.

Tap water is different in every area, and the only way to know what's in your water is to obtain a report from your local water facility. But tap water around the world has some things in common, like chlorine, which is necessary to disinfect it. Depending on where you are, tap water travels through miles and miles of waterlines, leaving it vulnerable to picking up contaminants along the way, possibly through runoff from farmland or industrial waste. According to the Environmental Working Group (EWG), nearly all water has an average of 300 contaminants of which half were not tested by the Environmental Protection Agency.

Bottled water may or may not be better. Most bottled waters are simply tap water that has been run through a carbon filter. Even if the water is of good quality, the bottles used often contain harmful chemicals that leach into the drinking water. And plastic bottles are simply bad for the environment as only 10-30% of them get recycled; the rest go into land-fills.

The cumulation of chemicals from tap water, certain bottled waters and their containers are stored in your body, and slowly leach into your system over time. These include chlorine, pesticides, fluorinated com-pounds, and plastics, which have been shown to interfere with the hu-man reproductive system. Unfortunately, these chemicals are found in both tap and bottled water and are known to interfere with hormone balance, something that you want to avoid, especially when you get older. If you have entered or passed menopause or are an older male, this still affects you because you still have a hormonal system that is susceptible to cancers and other chronic diseases.

Luckily, water filters have come to our rescue. A water treatment filter can make your water taste better, remove pathogens like giardia and e-coli, and remove chlorine, fluoride and other manmade contaminants like pesticides and metals. Water filters range from pitchers with a carbon filter to entire home filtration systems that will clean the water in all sinks, showers, bathtubs and refrigerators.

✓The Solution

Filter the water in your home to the extant that you are able to. For small spaces, a countertop water pitcher might be suitable, but for cleaner wa-ter look for water filters that fit right onto the tap, under the sink or for your entire home. If finances don't allow for the entire home, then at least filter your kitchen for drinking water and the bathroom where you brush your teeth and shower. The following guidelines can help you determine what type of filtration system to choose from.

- **Activated Carbon Filters** are the most popular and used in any type of filtration system. It helps remove chlorine, chloroform, agricultural contaminants and more.

- **Reverse Osmosis** effectively removes many manmade contaminants including fluoride, radium and arsenic, as well as pathogens. This is the most popular type of filter, but can cause low water pressure as the process is slow, and they tend to use a lot of water.

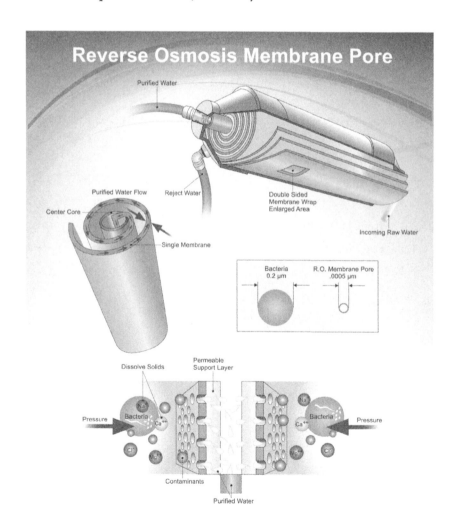

- **UV Filters** are used in some clinical situations because the ultraviolet light can kill bacteria and viruses. These are best used with activated carbon for a complete water cleaning.

Keep in mind that water pitchers with filters are mainly to help water smell and taste better, with an NSF/ANSI 42 certification being the standard. But if you want a water pitcher filter system that also removes contaminants, look for the NSF/ANSI 53 certification. In either case, make sure the pitcher material is made from BPA-free material.

Choosing a filtration system is dependent on where you live and the quality of the tap water. To help you learn about your region, the EWG has created a database you can find online called the Tap Water Database.

A human being would certainly not grow to be 70 or 80 years old if this longevity had no meaning for the species to which he belongs. The afternoon of human life must also have a significance of its own and cannot be merely a pitiful appendage to life's morning.

—Carl Jung

You can also find good quality mineral water that is sold in glass bottles, such as Perrier, Evian or San Pellegrino. Mineral water can help improve your skin, aid digestion, prevent osteoporosis and replenish electrolytes. These waters don't come cheap, especially when you're consuming them daily, but they definitely do provide numerous health benefits.

Overdrinking

For decades now we are repeatedly told to drink liters if not gallons of water for optimal health. I honestly bought right into this for many years and despite it feeling counterintuitive, I forced myself to drink way more than my body actually required. I truly believed that by the time you're thirsty, it's too late and you're on the brink of total dehydration. A few years ago, I started looking further into this and also realized that water has become a huge business.

Think back to when we were kids. Did everyone walk around with water bottles? Of course not! Nobody even sold bottled water back then. Not only that, but our parents didn't tell us to drink all the time and I don't recall anyone in my circle of friends who died of dehydration. Then I looked at animals. I have 3 dogs. Not once do I have to tell them when to drink nor how much. They drink when they're thirsty and they stop when they had enough. When did we lose this ability as humans? When did common sense just go out the window?

We are not victims of aging, sickness, and death. These are part of scenery, not the seer, who is immune to any form of change. This seer is the spirit, the expression of eternal being.

—**Deepak Chopra**

Overdrinking can actually cause major issues in your body. There is such a thing as water intoxication, a potentially fatal disturbance in brain functions that results when the normal balance of electrolytes in the body is pushed outside safe limits by excessive water intake. Over-hydration can lead to lower electrolyte levels, which can cause headaches, nausea, and muscle weakness. If your lips, hands, and feet are swollen, you may be consuming too much water.

✓The Solution

Think and live instinctively. Listen to your body. Drink when you're thirsty and drink until you feel satisfied. Obviously, your body will require more hydration during exercise or in hot weather, but there's no reason to force yourself to drink liters of water every day.

Please check out this video from Dr. Berg for more info:

Channel: Dr. Eric Berg DC
Drink 8 Glasses of Water Per Day - BIG FAT LIE! - Dr.Berg

The belief that youth is the happiest time of life is founded on a fallacy. The happiest person is the person who thinks the most interesting thoughts and we grow happier as we grow older.

—William Lyon Phelps

Coffee and Caffeinated Beverages

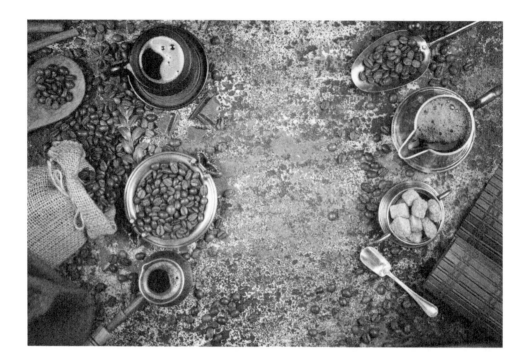

When it comes to aging gracefully, we might not consider our coffee habit. But quitting coffee, energy drinks and other caffeinated drinks can have some real anti-aging benefits. Some of these are as follows:

- You will experience improved sleep. Caffeine interferes with restorative sleep and your ability to fall asleep quickly.

- Your mood will improve, mainly because when you are not addicted to caffeine, you will not be grumpy before your first cup of coffee, and you won't feel lethargic in the afternoon as the caffeine wears off. And because caffeine stimulates the central nervous system, it can interfere with important neurotransmitters, leaving you open to irritability, anxiety and depression.

- Caffeine raises blood pressure in most people, and unfortunately this becomes worse as we age. Remember that caffeine is a drug that affects all bodily systems. When it causes a rise in blood pressure, it means your heart is working too hard. This is not the same as conditioning your heart with exercise.

- Coffee can stain your teeth, making them dingy, yellow and sometimes gray. This discoloration can be difficult to clean with regular brushing and might require a visit to the dentist for teeth whitening, if you want to keep your smile youthful.

- You might lose weight. For many people, coffee can add unnecessary calories through the added sugar and extra milk or cream. If you drink soy milk on a regular basis, you may become susceptible to belly bloat. Lastly, regular coffee use can cause the liver to become sluggish, which makes it more difficult to maintain a healthy weight.

- Your hormones will be more balanced. Caffeine raises stress hormones like cortisol, putting your body in a fight or flight mode every single day. Excess cortisol will age you more quickly and also signal to your body to store fat.

Check out my video for more info on coffee:

Channel: The Aging Games
Is Your Coffee Killing You? Why I Stopped Drinking Coffee

✓The Solution

The most obvious solution is to replace coffee with an herbal tea that contains no caffeine. But stopping abruptly might cause fatigue and headaches, so try replacing coffee with a tea that has a lower caffeine amount.

The more you drink coffee, the more your skin loses moisture. What happens when your skin loses its natural moisture? It loses its shine and glow and can lead to collagen loss and skin inflammation.

Some of these teas often come with health benefits and include green tea, oolong tea and white tea. Other teas to replace coffee with include Earl Grey and Chai tea, which also have herbs that are beneficial to your health.

Replace your morning coffee with dry skin brushing. This is an invigorating act that stimulates blood flow, lymphatic flow, removes dead skin cells and even stimulates your nervous system without drugs. Simply use a brush with natural bristles created for this purpose, and using short, quick strokes begin at your feet, and work your way up the body, always brushing toward your heart. It should take no more that 2—3 minutes.

Exercise as soon as you get out of bed. If you work or have other morning commitments, set your alarm clock for 15 minutes earlier. Choose from exercises like taking a walk, get a rebounder and jump in the morning, or get a yoga DVD and use it. By the time you are done, you will no longer have a need for coffee.

Decaf can be a good alternative if you enjoy the taste and ritual of having coffee. Look for Swiss Water Decaf coffee that is decaffeinated without the use of chemicals.

I believe the second half of one's life is meant to be better than the first half. The first half is finding out how you do it. And the second half is enjoying it.

—**Frances Lear**

Deuterium Depleted Water

What is Deuterium Depleted Water?

Deuterium is called heavy water (D20)
Unlike hydrogen with a single proton,
 deuterium contains a neutron in it's nucleus.

Most water contains about 150 ppm of D2O.

DEUTERIUM

Deuterium affects electron chain transport in the mitochondria, ATP production is slowed and unusual free radical signals are made. A body with a high amount of deuterium will experience impaired vitamin D production, and higher heteroplasmy rates, leading to earlier death and disease.

Water in cold climates contains less deuterium than water in warmer climates. Winter precipitation contains less deuterium than summer precipitation. Water at high altitudes has less deuterium.

Studies have shown drinking deuterium depleted water (25-125ppm) helps restore immune function, reverse cancer, and stop mtDNA damage.

vigr.ca

Deuterium depleted water (DDW) is water that has no deuterium, which is a hydrogen molecule that contains an extra particle. Most water contains one deuterium molecule for every 3,200 regular water molecules. All animal bodies are about 75% water, and so all will contain some deuterium, including humans. Humans, animals, plants, and other living creatures can deplete deuterium naturally when they are young and healthy, but this changes as we get older. So, why would we want to deplete deuterium from our bodies?

Our cells and the mitochondria within the cells, along with gut flora have the ability to detox deuterium through natural bodily functions like breathing, sweating and urinating. Living organisms need these molecules, but must keep levels in check because high levels of deuterium become toxic. As with many other bodily functions, as we get older, our deuterium depletion abilities seem to lessen.

> "If you associate enough with older people who do enjoy their lives, who are not stored away in any golden ghettos, you will gain a sense of continuity and of the possibility for a full life.
>
> —**Margaret Mead**

Deuterium instigates a slower reaction rate in mitochondria than standard hydrogen atoms. In other words, deuterium slows down chemical reactions, which may be a problem in some bodily functions. Because of this, medical researchers have been investigating the effects of DDW on cancer cells and tumors. Surprisingly, they have found "convincing empirical evidence" that DDW has an anticancer effect.[5] In other words, it either slows the growth of or outright eliminates cancer cells! Other studies show it may help treat obesity, and may have a positive effect on glucose metabolism, as well.

Too much deuterium in the body can lead to mitochondrial dysfunction, which translates to immunity issues, metabolic problems and premature aging. As you help your body remove excess deuterium through lifestyle changes, your body can more easily repair itself. When the body repairs

---

5   Zhang X, Gaetani M, Chernobrovkin A, Zubarev RA. Anticancer Effect of Deuterium Depleted Water - Redox Disbalance Leads to Oxidative Stress. Mol Cell Proteomics. 2019;18(12):2373-2387. doi:10.1074/mcp.RA119.001455

itself, it not only repairs what is damaged, like a broken wrist, but it constantly repairs and replaces worn out cells in the muscles, skin and hair. When your body is more efficient at this process, the aging process slows down.

✓ The Solution

We can naturally reduce deuterium in the body through diet. In fact, a low-carb, whole food diet results in lower deuterium levels in the body as opposed to a diet high in processed foods. Fat and meat from grass-fed animals is the most profound deuterium depleted food source around. Adopting a diet high in fat like a natural paleo-ketogenic diet can help your body produce your own deuterium depleted water inside your cells, hydrating your body from the inside out. This may be because food processing removes the naturally low-level deuterium plant components from the whole foods, leaving behind "heavier" molecules. In addition, industrial food preparation often involves periods of high intensity heat resulting in evaporation of much of the natural water, leaving behind a concentration of deuterium in the food.

Aside from sticking with a wholesome diet, many have found quicker success by using Deuterium Depleted Water (DDW), which is water that has either less or no deuterium content. While water that is completely free of deuterium is only found in the polar regions, water with lower amounts is more readily available. According to those who work in the health industry, drinking water with 125 to 136 ppm (parts per million) can potentially slow the aging process. This type of water comes from glaciers and other cold regions and is fairly affordable. Regular tap water normally contains 150 ppm or higher; another reason to avoid tap water.

Other ways to reduce deuterium in your body include fasting, cold thermogenesis and exercise, but more about those later.

Depleting deuterium may boost your energy production and repair your mitochondria, and could be a great way to lose unwanted body fat and to slow down the aging process.

EZ Water and Your Mitochondria

Brought to light by scientist Dr. Gerald Pollack, EZ water stands for Exclusion Zone water, and designates a type of water found in certain parts of a cell where the "water" is more of a gel or membrane. Also called structured water, EZ water is like a charged battery that has the power to deliver energy to your cells. It also strengthens your mitochondria so you can produce more energy. Water is a known conduit and helps send messages throughout all the cells in your body, including messages of healing or sickness. Just like radio waves or any other type of wave, negative messages often result in negative outcomes.

The idea of helping your body create more, healthy EZ water within your cells stems from science that finds certain water is healthier than the water that is bottled in plastic and stored for months, or water that is simply run through miles of pipelines and treated with chemicals; both are unnatural way to consume water.

But by consuming the "right" type of water, you can help your body create more of the healthy structured water to better deliver nutritional or health messages throughout your cells. EZ water helps your body and cells literally generate more energy, which in turn helps proteins repair while cellular aging slows. The result is more energy so your body can more efficiently ward off the aging process, accelerate healing and recovery, fight stress and supercharge your brain. And while the science is new and growing, the health practices that can help us accomplish this have withstood the test of time.

✓The Solution

Structured water is found in many places throughout nature. In addition, with the right nutritional tools, our bodies can more readily make it. The following are some solutions to help you take advantage of this wonderful anti-aging gift that nature has to offer.

When it comes to staying young, a mind-lift beats a face-lift any day."

—Marty Buccella

- Spring water, unadulterated, and from natural source becomes structured as is it deep in the ground and under pressure. If you have a source near you, that can be your water source. You can also buy good quality spring water in glass bottles.

- Like plants, the human body not only needs water but also sunlight. The near-infrared rays in sunlight penetrate deep into your skin and structure the water in your cells. Naked sunbathing provides the type of light that your body can use to create internal EZ water. It forms when skin is exposed to natural sunlight without the filter of sunscreen, clothing or sunglasses. Sun exposure plays a crucial role in your body's energy production. Your cells actually act as "light-driven batteries." (Another reason not to fear the sun!)

- Infrared saunas are a way to receive a concentrated dose of infrared light, which helps your body make its own EZ water. Some researchers believe this is why IR saunas are effective at accelerating muscle recovery after a workout.

- Turmeric, coconut water, coconut oil and ghee have all been found by Pollack's team to increase EZ in your cells.

EZ water fights aging and stress and helps your body recover faster. It's the ultimate anti-aging tool.

- Grounding/Earthing - by walking barefoot on the ground or sand or by swimming in the sea you absorb negatively charged ions from the Earth, which helps build EZ

- Add an ionic mineral solution to your drinking water. The mineral in these types of solutions is black mica, or biotite, and a few drops purifies water and helps it become structured water.

- Eat more animal fat. Your body can produce 110 grams of metabolic water per 100 grams of fat eaten.

Drinking enough water will not always hydrate you. There are plenty of individuals who drink their 6 to 8 glasses a day and do not appear any more hydrated than those who don't. But when you drink the 'right' water, your body can better use it, meaning it can get into your cells and where it's needed for hydration, recharging and healing. You will feel and see the difference, and the solutions are not difficult to incorporate into your daily schedule.

Consume Bone Broth

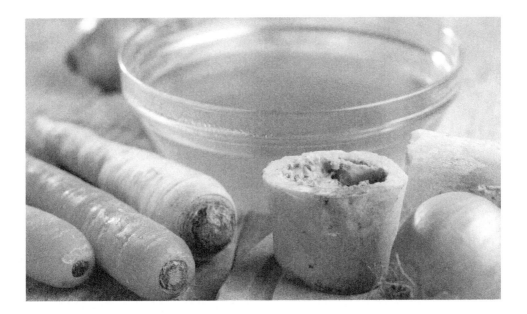

Bone broth is making a resurgence in the kitchens of health advocates around the world. For centuries, it was common to keep a kettle cooking 24 hours a day, and in this kettle unused plant parts and bones from the tribal hunt were deposited and allowed to simmer. The tradition was to be grateful for everything and to waste nothing that was provided for your family and tribe. It has also been a staple in Traditional Chinese Medicine (TCM) for thousands of years. And today, we know that the broth was not just a way to ensure nothing goes to waste, but is an incredible functional food for healing and antiaging!

Bone broth is a broth or stock made with vegetables, herbs, bones and cartilage of animals. The healthiest are from grass fed, free range animals, as opposed to commercially farmed ones. It's rich in minerals, collagen and amino acids, and so promotes healing in the digestive tract, strengthens joints and bones, strengthens the immune system and even helps the body manufacture collagen for youthful firmness and elasticity.

My physical body may be less efficient and less beautiful in old age. But God has given me an enormous compensation: my mind is richer my Soul is broader and my wisdom is at a peak. I am so happy with the riches of my advanced peak age that, contrary to Faust, I would not wish to return to youth.

—Robert Muller

Some in the medical industry claim that your body will not use collagen for the skin, because since it is a form of protein, the body will break it down into amino acids and use it elsewhere. However, at least one study using a specific oral liquid collagen supplement did show participants experienced a significant improvement in skin elasticity and hydration. The body was able to synthesize the collagen protein, meaning that "age-dependent reduction" in collagen synthesis can be reversed.[6]

Other smaller studies showed that bone broth can make your joints and bones stronger, and that it can improve symptoms such as joint pain and stiffness in people with osteoarthritis. If it can do that, then it may be able to help most people with pain and stiffness that seems to accompany age. No matter what benefits you desire to see, whether it's less pain, youthful skin or better digestion and metabolism, the key is in the quality.

Bone broth is not the same as beef broth or chicken broth. Bone broth is made by slowly simmering bones on low heat over a long period of time, allowing the bone marrow, collagen and other nutritional components to break down and infiltrate the liquid. For this reason, the most nutritious forms will be from free range animals. Free range, grass fed protein is superior and always considered a more nutritious source of healthy fats

---

6   Bolke L, Schlippe G, Gerß J, Voss W. A Collagen Supplement Improves Skin Hydration, Elasticity, Roughness, and Density: Results of a Randomized, Placebo-Controlled, Blind Study. Nutrients. 2019;11(10):2494. Published 2019 Oct 17. doi:10.3390/nu11102494

and minerals and is a more humane practice with fewer toxins than factory farms induce.

✓The Solution

If you would like to add bone broth into your weekly diet, many natural food stores carry the healthier versions. How much one should drink depends upon your individual nutritional needs, but most experts claim anywhere from 1 to 4 cups per day. The following recipes can help you make your own.

Save bones from a whole, free range, organic chicken or bones from a roast or other beef (3-4 pounds), or roast raw bones. You can often get bones from your butcher for free as they get discarded. Add enough spring water to cover the bones along with about 2 Tablespoons of apple cider vinegar and let sit for 30 minutes. Add any chopped vegetables if you like, such as onion, carrots, fennel, etc. and herbs such as garlic, rosemary or peppercorns. Bring to a boil, then lower to a simmer. Clear off and dispose of any foam that develops on the surface. Most broth can be simmered for 24 hours, while larger bones can simmer for 48 hours. If you don't want to leave a pot on the stovetop, use an oven pot on very low heat or a slow cooker.

| Water Fasting

Fasting with water is an age-old practice for health and religious reasons. It involves simply refraining from eating or drinking anything except for pure, clean spring water for a day or more. The practice has numerous health

Bone broth is said to improve skin quality and promote elasticity and help the skin stay wrinkle-free and youthful.

benefits, and reviews of medical studies show various periods of water fasting are associated with lower metabolic disease markers, wards of dementia and Alzheimer's disease, helps with long-term memory, lessens depressive episodes and is the most effective way to lower hypertension.[7] Together, this makes water fasting sound like the perfect anti-aging gift. But there is a catch.

One cannot simply begin water fasting, because it can lead to serious symptoms that might harm certain people, especially if you have a medical condition. Therefore, if you want to try it, get the okay from your doctor, first. Then understand there are numerous ways to water fast.

One practice is to fast by drinking water only one to two days every week, without eating any food. This is done by some religious groups and has been shown to considerably reduce the risk of heart disease. The length of time and frequency of your fasts will determine your results. To get the most out of your fast, prepare your body ahead of time.

Check out my video about water fasting:

> Channel: The Aging Games
> How to Lose Weight with Water Fasting in 10 Days?

✓ The Solution

If you began fasting tomorrow without any preparation, chances are you will feel either sick or lethargic and then energetic by day two and so on. It is normal to cycle in and out of feeling good and bad, but for

---

7   de Cabo R, Carmona-Gutierrez D, Bernier M, Hall MN, Madeo F. The search for antiaging interventions: from elixirs to fasting regimens. Cell. 2014;157(7):1515-1526. doi:10.1016/j.cell.2014.05.031

all your hard work, the results should last, and those that prepare their bodies have longer lasting effects than those who don't.

Prepare your body by stopping junk and processed foods. Abstain from caffeine, alcohol, sugary treats, breads and all sodas. Replace one or two meals each day with bone broth to slowly prep your body for the fast. Allow at least a few days like this before you begin. If you're in ketosis when you begin your water fast, the process will be much easier as you will be less hungry.

Start your first water fast with just 24 hours. Sip on fresh spring water throughout the day. Add a bit of pink salt, especially if you're feeling dizzy or feel a headache coming on. Take a relaxing bath, but not too hot, add essential oils, and enjoy the healing process. Do not exercise and try to keep your activity levels low. If you are experienced at fasting, aim for longer, but stop if you feel too lightheaded, dizzy, or any side effects that feel dangerous. Recruit the aid of a health practitioner or doctor if you can, for safety reasons, and be sure to tell family members what you are doing, especially if you live alone.

When done right, you will experience the amazing benefits of water fasting. More energy is usually the first benefit that people report. Regular water fasting can also help with weight loss efforts and fix a sluggish metabolism.

Break your fast slowly with some bone broth, kefir, or yogurt.

New research has found that fasting triggers a molecule that can delay the aging of our arteries. The findings could help prevent age-related chronic diseases such as cancer, cardiovascular disease, and Alzheimer's.

Fat Fasting

Fat fasting is loosely based on the popular low-carb, high-fat diets and is designed to be performed from 2 to 5 days. During this time, you consume 1,000 to 1,200 calories per day and 80% to 90% of calories should be from fat. This is not true "fasting," but a technique used to quickly shed a few pounds, to break a weight loss plateau or to kick start your body into ketosis; the state where fat is burned for energy instead of carbohydrates.

By totally eliminating carbohydrates, your body begins to burn fat as fuel and the fat your body uses is not just from the food you are consuming. If you can get your body into ketosis, which this "fast" is designed to do, your body burns fat as its source of energy. As we get older, hormonal changes can lead to weight gain, while muscles atrophy and body fat increases. This fat fast can be the hack that gets you out of the aging cycle so you can head into a healthier fitness plan and experience real results.

My experience with Fat Fasting here:

Channel: The Aging Games
Fat Fasting | Fasting Mimicking Diet Keto Style

✓The Solution

Plan your meals for 2 to 5 days, depending on how long you will fast. If this is your first time, your goal should be no longer than 3 days.

Your choice of foods should include fatty but healthy foods like avocado, macadamia nuts, full fat cream and high-fat cheese. Small amounts of protein can include grass fed beef, bacon, or chicken (dark meat and skin). Add-ons can include mayonnaise, herbs, ghee, lard, bone broth, coconut oil, sour cream, dairy butter and nut butters.

Find recipes online to cover 3-5 meals a day. Meals and snacks are similar to these:

Fat fasting will force the body to undergo lipolysis so that it burns up fat that is stored in the body.

- Egg and bacon filled baked avocados

- 1 ounce macadamia nuts with cream cheese

- 1 celery stalk with 2 ounces of cream cheese

- 3 bacon slices with 2 egg yolks

- 1 cup bone broth with 2 tbsp heavy cream

- Classic buffalo wings with sugar free ranch dressing

- Egg Muffins made with scrambled eggs, chopped bacon, cheese, green onion and red pepper bits baked in muffin tins

The key is to limit protein and cut out carbohydrates, so your body relies only on fat for energy. If you were not in ketosis when you started it might be an uncomfortable two or three days, but keep in mind it's what is known as the "keto flu" and it will pass. Be sure to drink spring or filtered water to help your body remove metabolic waste.

It should be noted that this fast may not be for everyone. If you have gallbladder issues, the fat intake can cause issues. For some, this technique may cause fluctuations in blood sugar, heartbeat and blood pressure. If you take any medications or have any medical conditions, either talk to your doctor or skip this one, altogether.

Intermittent Fasting and OMAD

OMAD stands for One Meal A Day, and I put it with intermittent fasting (IF) as they are very similar. The concept of one meal a day is self-explanatory, while IF involves eating a few meals but within a set number of hours. The most popular time frame is to eat during an eight-hour window, and then fast for 16 hours. For example, you can eat from 8am until 4pm, then fast until 8am the next day.

With OMAD people are having just one meal a day, within a one-hour window and then fast again for almost 24 hours.

When it comes to weight loss, many people have success with IF by allowing a 4- to 6-hour window to eat, which creates a longer fasting time. Other ways to do IF are to eat a healthy, wholesome diet for 5 days a week, then fast for 2, or to alternate one day of eating with one day of fasting. But why would anyone want to do this, and what does it have to do with how we age?

Evidence is mounting that shows intermittent fasting helps trigger anti-aging effects, including the stimulation of HGH, or human growth hormone. This is one of our most important anti-aging hormones as it helps build bone and muscle mass, assists in the firmness of our skin, and boosts metabolism. It also helps us recover after exercise and speeds healing of an injury. And it helps the brain maintain and build healthy tissue and more easily repair it when needed.

Studies not only show that fasting stimulates growth hormone, but it can help your brain clear away unwanted, used up proteins and other debris.[8] The process is called neuronal autophagy, meaning the brain has the ability to detoxify itself, and some researchers believe short bouts

---

8   Alirezaei M, Kemball CC, Flynn CT, Wood MR, Whitton JL, Kiosses WB. Short-term fasting induces profound neuronal autophagy. Autophagy. 2010;6(6):702-710. doi:10.4161/auto.6.6.12376

of fasting are a safe and simple method to stimulate the process.

Other important benefits of IF that contribute to anti aging include increased cellular repair throughout the entire body, as well as autophagy as described above, but for the whole body. Also, this type of fasting leads to healthy changes in genes that are linked to disease prevention and longevity.

Check out my video about OMAD:

> Channel: The Aging Games
> 5 Benefits of OMAD | One Meal a Day Diet for Weight Loss

Autophagy is the most powerful tool that we have when it comes to anti-aging. It is your body's own technique for spring cleaning. It eliminates the cells that are damaged and no longer functional.

✓The Solution

Intermittent Fasting is not just a new buzzword in the diet world but a true gem when it comes to weight loss and anti-aging. You can try IF by limiting the window within which you have your meals. You can start with the most popular one 16/8—where you're fasting for 16 hours and eating within an 8-hour window. The earlier you have your last meal during the day, the more effective this will be. Once you've gotten used to this way of eating, you can shorten your eating window to 6, 4 and eventually even give OMAD a try.

Consume Less Carbohydrates

Consuming less carbs sounds like part of the low-carb diet, but this practice should be done no matter if you are on a low-carb diet or not. When it comes to aging, certain types of carbohydrates actually accelerate the aging process. This is because when carbs are converted into sugar, it damages a component of our DNA called telomeres, which quickens the death of the telomere while damaging the DNA strand. The quicker our DNA strands become damaged, the quicker we age. Now let's talk about the worst kinds of carbs.

> "
>
> I'm baffled that anyone might not think women get more beautiful as they get older. Confidence comes with age, and looking beautiful comes from the confidence someone has in themselves.
>
> **—Kate Winslet**

White flour, like in white bread and pasta, has a direct effect on our bodies. It has a high glycemic index, which means it not only causes a jump in blood sugar, but can stimulate chronic internal inflammation, a condition linked to age-related diseases like diabetes and heart disease. It also causes weight gain, which most of us can do without.

Refined carbs are the biggest aging culprits in many people's diets. White flour is one of these, but also cookies, cakes, bakery items, certain cereals, processed rice and anything made with white flour. These are all highly processed with added chemicals and preservatives. The good news is that you can easily replace carbs with healthier options.

✓The Solution

- Try some healthy Keto bread recipes to replace the bread in your diet

- Slowly get used to not having bread with meals (this takes some getting used to)

- Replace breakfast cereals with healthy proteins and fat. This will help sustain you for much longer than sugary cereals.

- Replace the highly processed white rice with wild rice, wheat berries or buckwheat, and be sure to keep the portion very small.

- If you have a sweet tooth, replace treats with plain Greek yogurt with added stevia and blueberries or strawberries.

Foods with a high glycemic index, like white bread, can cause inflammation in the body, which is directly linked to the aging process.

None are so old as those who have outlived enthusiasm.

—Henry David Thoreau

Eliminate Sugar

Sugar harms the body and accelerates aging like nothing else. For those who desire to take care of their health and maintain health and energy while warding off the aging process, eliminating sugar from your diet can make a huge impact.

Many foods, drinks and condiments can be okay in moderation for some people. The problem with sugar is that there is just so much of it in everything we drink and eat. It is added to breads, cereals, fruit juice, soups, cured meats, deli meats, and condiments. Sodas, sweetened teas and fruit juices can have three times the daily recommended amount and more. Many people add it to coffee or tea (among other things) and may indulge in an occasional dessert, adding onto the daily sugar they most likely didn't realize they had already consumed.

Grow old along with me!
The best is yet to be.

—Robert Browning

The average American adult consumes more than three times the recommended limit for sugar intake. Sugar consumption in the United States (and worldwide) has been on the rise in the past decade. Between 2018 and 2019, Americans consumed about 11 million metric tons of sugar, up from about 10 million metric tons in 2010. According to government statistics, the average American consumes almost 152 pounds (almost 70kg) of sugar in one year. This is equal to 3 pounds (or 6 cups) of sugar consumed every week.

Consuming high amounts of sugar increases your risk of dying from heart disease. According to a study published in the Journal of the American Medical Association (JAMA), one 15-year study found that those who got just 17% of their caloric intake from sugar had a 38% increased risk of dying from heart disease.[9]

Added sugar is also responsible for high obesity rates. That's because sugar is addictive and makes you crave more. In fact, it follows the same additive neuropathways that cocaine does. Along with obesity, it greatly increases your risk for diabetes and cancer. As we get older, we should aim to lower our risk factors, and learning to live without sugar is one of the best things you can do for your body.

Sugar contributes to 35 million deaths a year worldwide, according to researchers from the University of California.

✓The Solution

- Keep track of your sugar intake. You might be shocked at how much more you're consuming than you thought.

- Read labels for hidden sugars, or avoid processed foods altogether.

- Exchange dessert for a small piece of low-carb fruit or make after dinner herbal tea a habit.

- Use Stevia or honey as an occasional sweetener.

- Detoxify your body.

- Practice abstinence from all sugars to help your body detox it. You might experience withdrawal effects like depression and headaches, so talk to your doctor, if necessary. Keep in mind that this, too, shall pass.

---

9   Publishing, H. (n.d.). The sweet danger of sugar. Retrieved October 30, 2020, from **https://www.health.harvard.edu/heart-health/the-sweet-danger-of-sugar**

Eliminate Artificial Sweeteners

I thought I should add this after the sugar section, because artificial sweeteners are the replacement that most people think of when quitting sugar. Artificial sweeteners are promoted to help reduce the risks associated with too much sugar consumption, which includes diabetes, heart disease and metabolic syndrome. But artificial sweeteners have their own set of issues, which are no friend to anti-aging.

The wiser mind mourns less for what age takes away than what it leaves behind.

—William Wordsworth

The main culprits include aspartame, saccharin, sucralose, neotame and acesulfame. Mainstream scientists and nutritionists warn of consuming more calories to replace the lack of sugar, or that the sweeteners can stimulate sugar cravings, leading to bingeing. But there are worse concerns than these.

One example is the effect of aspartame on cell life. According to neurosurgeon Russell Blaylock, aspartame is one of a set of neurotoxins that stimulates brain cells to death, resulting in premature cell death and thus, aging. Studies that show sweeteners like these are "safe" do not test with the more than 24 ounces of sweetened beverages that are consumed on average.

One study showed that diet drink consumption was linked to a 36% increased risk of metabolic syndrome and 67% increased risk for type 2 diabetes, making these artificially sweetened drinks no better than their sugar-laden counterparts.[10] This may be because artificial sweeteners

---

10   Strawbridge, H. (2020, February 03). Artificial sweeteners: Sugar-free, but at what cost? Retrieved October 30, 2020, from **https://www.health.harvard.edu/blog/artificial-sweeteners-sugar-free-but-at-what-cost-201207165030**

increase blood glucose, and constant consumption leads to chronically high blood sugar, which causes the signs of aging like wrinkles and other skin conditions as well as age-related disease.

✓ The Solution

Stevia is the one, true sweetener that can be safe in small doses. It is made from the extracts of the green leaves of the plant, resulting in steviol glycosides. This makes stevia up to 300 times sweeter than white, table sugar, so be careful how much you use. Also, because it has become a popular sugar substitute, read the labels to see if the product is pure stevia. Some brands add synthetic chemicals to save money, so you could be getting a combination of stevia mixed with aspartame or another of the sweeteners that are unhealthy. And keep in mind that stevia is still a sweetener and processed, so use it in moderation.

Another thing to consider is that even though stevia and other natural sweeteners have little effect on your blood sugar level, they still have an effect on your insulin level, and a lot of people who struggle with weight issues are insulin resistant. So even though stevia doesn't contain many calories, it can still stimulate insulin, which leads to weight gain.

The best solution and alternative to artificial sweeteners is to learn to live without consuming sweets. Try water infused with mint, cucumber and lemon or herbal teas alone. Your tastebuds will adjust and then you can save money and your skin by simply going all natural.

High insulin levels are the main cause of hormonal imbalances and many skin disorders. Since artificial sweeteners throw your blood sugar balance off, they can cause premature aging.

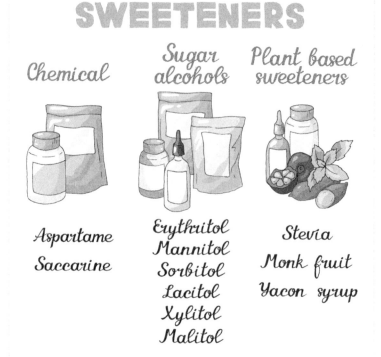

SWEETENERS

Chemical

Aspartame
Saccarine

Sugar alcohols

Erythritol
Mannitol
Sorbitol
Lacitol
Xylitol
Malitol

Plant based sweeteners

Stevia
Monk fruit
Yacon syrup

Choose Healthy Cooking Oils

In spite of what the mainstream science tells us, vegetables oils, even canola and sunflower, are not healthy sources for our healthy fats. The "evidence" that the National Institutes of Health, the American Heart Association and other institutes has been based on incomplete date going back to the 1960s, in which they believed that replacing saturated fats (like butter) with vegetable oil (like corn oil) led to lower cholesterol therefore less heart disease. Until they found a "lost" study from Michigan that showed in spite of the lowered cholesterol those who used corn oil to replace butter had a great risk of dying from heart disease.[11]

To date, no institute has turned around and looked at the "new" evidence, while millions of people continue to listen to bad science. There are many reasons for this from lack of funding to lack of interest, but the lesson to learn is that vegetable oils are poison to the body. Here's why…

Getting old is like climbing a mountain; you get a little out of breath, but the view is much better!

—Ingrid Bergman

Vegetables oils like corn, canola, sunflower, soybean and safflower are highly unstable. Unstable molecules are known to be highly inflammatory, meaning they create internal inflammation in our bodies. This condition is linked to accelerated aging and chronic disease. This may be because they are high in Omega 6, which isn't necessarily bad if it is balanced with the appropriate amount of Omega 3s. As I already mentioned, the average person consumes about 20 times more Omega 6s than they should, and this balance (or lack of balance) can kill you.

✓The Solution

Stick to natural, saturated fats that our ancestors ate for thousands of years. Lard is one of the healthiest, containing 60% of monounsaturated fats, which is linked to lowered heart disease. You probably didn't see this coming, right? Your grandma was right all along! Oleic acid is the type of fat found in lard, which is the same substance that makes olive oil healthy. Lard has a high cooking point, meaning you can cook with

---

11   Replacing butter with vegetable oils does not cut heart disease risk. (2016, April 12). Retrieved October 30, 2020, from https://www.sciencedaily.com/releases/2016/04/160412211335.htm

You would have to eat 98 ears of corn in order to consume five tablespoons of corn oil.

it and your food will not become carcinogenic. The same cannot be said for vegetable oils and even olive oil should not be used for frying.

Butter and ghee are runner ups following lard, with 45% monounsaturated fats. And if you use grass-fed butter, you will get even more health benefits including vitamins A and K2, both good for bone and heart health.

Don't Eat After Sundown

While this may not be a nutritional aspect of diet, it is an important component worth mentioning. Our digestion is one of many bodily functions that work on a 24-hour cycle. This cycle happens to peak in the middle of the day and becomes weaker as the day goes on. By nighttime, it comes close to hibernation as it slows through the night. We can eat at night, but that does not guarantee your digestive enzymes will wake up and begin to work.

Interestingly, in the ancient Indian religion or philosophy of Jain Dharma, eating at night is prohibited. The belief is that harmful microbes that are easily destroyed by the sun come out of hiding at night, and thus, food becomes unhealthy. It is also believed that the "digestive fire" performs along with the sunrise and sunset, which is true as our enzymes are most active around noon when the sun is at its peak!

Studies have found that a same meal eaten at dinner as lunch time will raise blood sugar levels more in the evening than earlier in the day. This is even true for low-carb meals. If you are watching your weight, suffer from diabetes or digestive issues, it's even more important to not eat after sunset.

✓ Solution

Incorporating this practice might be difficult if you are traditionally a late eater or enjoy nighttime snacking. Luckily, it doesn't take long to break this habit, if you replace snacking with other activities like an evening yoga stretch or reading. If you are used to eating late, or your family does, try either influencing the family to eat earlier and explain the health reasons, or change your own mealtime to earlier. You can have tea with your family, or include a smaller meal, which is easier to digest than a full meal.

According to Dr. Jack Kruse, "when you eat post sunset your liver gets larger and you get leptin resistant and this causes metabolic changes in the leptin receptor in your hypothalamus."

Aging is not lost youth but a new stage of opportunity and strength.

—**Betty Friedan**

CHAPTER 4

Natural Supplements & Home Remedies

Home remedies have been part of daily health since the beginning of time. In fact, many medical treatments of today are based on herbal remedies of the past, and the practice continues to this day. In this section, some home remedies that are directly related to how we age will be presented. This is not an exhaustive list, but those listed here are easy enough and innovative enough to include in this book. As always, please check with your medical provider before taking supplements, especially if you're on medications.

Vitamin D to Reverse Aging

Of course, we need a variety of nutrients for overall health, but some that act as an excellent tool for anti-aging can easily become neglected in our daily diets. One example is vitamin D, a fat-soluble vitamin that is highly beneficial for your immune system and to reverse aging. The primary source of vitamin D is our own bodies, but we need the rays of the sun to make it happen. At the same time, we need to consume foods to ensure we get enough, because as we get older, our bodies become less capable of making this essential vitamin. The following are some reasons we cannot miss out on this all-important nutrient:

Strong Bones - One of the most important roles of vitamin D when it comes to aging is its impact on calcium absorption and bone health. It seems to help the bones repair and heal, and may even slow bone loss for those who have osteoporosis.

Weight Control - Weight management becomes more difficult as we age. But vitamin D stimulates the metabolism and can help curb blood sugar. In fact, one Italian study found that women who were overweight lost more weight when they supplemented with vitamin D than those

Vitamin D is crucial for women in midlife, as it may also play a role in moderating several perimenopausal and menopausal symptoms. Menopausal women are at higher risk of osteoporosis due to the lack of estrogen.

who did not take this vitamin, in spite of following the same diet.[1]

Longevity—Vitamin D interacts with what are known as "longevity genes," which can extend lifespan and slow age-related protein "mis-foldings." Proteins are found throughout the body and are responsible for tissue repair in every area from muscle building to brain healing. Proteins are known to "fold" into a functional shape, so they can then be used where needed by the body. When we age, proteins might "misfold," leading to tissue degeneration and disease. Luckily, vitamin D helps proteins to hold their shape and thus retain function for longer.

Immunity - Vitamin D can also act as a hormone in the body and help improve your immune system. This means less age-related immune system problems that tend to occur as we get older. This may be why this nutrient is linked to helping reduce the risk of breast and colon cancers.

Hair Health—Women who have higher blood levels of vitamin D experience significantly less hair loss than those with lower levels. Apparently, this vitamin is necessary for your body to create hair follicles, which allows new hair growth to take place.

✓The Solution

Most experts advise we need from 5 to 30 minutes of uninhibited sun exposure from three to seven days a week

1   Khosravi ZS, Kafeshani M, Tavasoli P, Zadeh AH, Entezari MH. Effect of Vitamin D Supplementation on Weight Loss, Glycemic Indices, and Lipid Profile in Obese and Overweight Women: A Clinical Trial Study. Int J Prev Med. 2018;9:63. Published 2018 Jul 20. doi:10.4103/ijpvm.IJPVM_329_15

for healthy synthesis of vitamin D. This means sun exposure on our face, arms, legs, and hands without sunblock.

Supplementing with vitamin D is an option for those who simply cannot get outside for their daily dose of sunshine or live in latitudes, where the UV exposure is not strong enough. Experts recommended using from 800 to 1,000 IU of vitamin D daily. Food sources of vitamin D include mushrooms, egg yolks, fatty fish, liver and other red meat.

Vitamin C Delays the Signs of Aging

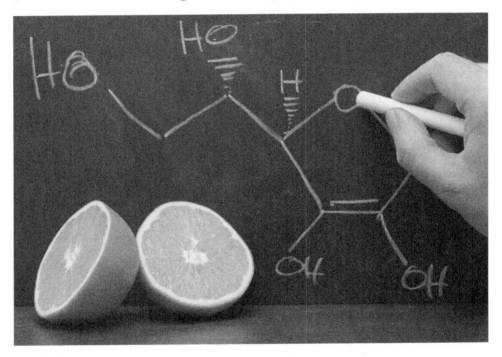

There's a reason why many beauty products use vitamin C in their creams and serums. This vitamin is needed for the production of collagen, which can help delay the signs of aging. Collagen is the network of protein fibers in the skin that helps keep it firm and elastic. It is also found in ligaments, tendons, bones and internal organs, and keeps these parts of our bodies strong as it provides strength and structure. It also works like a protective covering for the organs.

As we get older, collagen breaks down, which can lead to sagging skin, slow wound healing, and sluggish replacement of dead skin cells, among other things. Sadly, with age, collagen production slows down too, especially in post-menopausal women. As the skin's integrity declines with age, joint cartilage weakens, leaving us with sore knees or hips. Wrinkles form on the skin as it can no longer bounce back from stress.

> Anyone who stops learning is old, whether at twenty or eighty. Anyone who keeps learning stays young. The greatest thing in life is to keep your mind young.
>
> **—Henry Ford**

Vitamin C is important to help our bodies continue its production of collagen, but it has other anti-aging functions, as well. It is a powerful antioxidant that protects our cells from free radical damage. When left unchecked, free radicals are known to increase the risk of getting cancer. They are also involved in the aging process, and if oxidative stress takes over, your body will age prematurely. *Oxidative stress is a state where there are too many free radicals and not enough antioxidants to keep them in check.*

Vitamin C is such an important nutrient for anti-aging that it is used extensively in dermatologists' offices for various treatments. Some use it during microneedling procedures to treat scaring, hyperpigmentation, and for collagen synthesis. Professional grade skin peels include vitamin C for skin repair and renewal of the cells and to boost collagen. Besides using it topically, it is important to ensure you get plenty in your diet to help your body maintain protein and collagen synthesis throughout.

✓ The Solution

Because our bodies don't manufacture vitamin C, it is important to get it through diet. Since it is a water-soluble vitamin, your body cannot store it, so you have to consume it daily. Please remember to choose organic produce when possible for its higher nutritional value. Some top foods for vitamin C include:

In the absence of carbohydrates in one's diet, far less Vitamin C is needed, as it doesn't have to constantly compete with glucose for uptake.

- Citrus fruits
- Cantaloupe
- Red and green peppers
- Cauliflower
- Strawberries
- Tomatoes
- Brussel sprouts
- Spinach

As with any nutrient, if you feel you need a supplement, look for those that are from whole food sources. Studies have found Ester-C® to be better absorbed and excreted less rapidly than ascorbic acid and to have superior scurvy-preventing activity.

DHA and EPA

DHA and EPA are both healthy fats from the Omega-3 class. Docosahexaenoic acid (DHA) supports brain health, vision and heart health, while eicosapentaenoic acid (EPA) also supports brain health and lowers the risk of heart disease.

The health benefits of these fatty acids are mainly found when combined, which means they seem to complement each other. This is especially true for heart and brain health, and when used together they create powerful protection as they help reduce inflammation and help arteries remain elastic. This in turn helps lower blood pressure, keeps your blood flowing freely and reduces your risk of heart disease.

Here's what I know: I'm a better person at fifty than I was at forty-eight … and better at fifty-two than I was at fifty. I'm calmer, easier to live with. All this stuff is in my soul forever. Just don't get lazy. Work at your relationships all the time. Take care of friendships, hold people you love close to you, take advantage of birthdays to celebrate fiercely. It's the worrying — not the years themselves — that will make you less of a woman.

—Patti LaBelle

Our brains rely on healthy fatty acids. In fact, more research today shows that people who regularly consume foods that are rich in omega-3 fats can help ward of dementia and Alzheimer's disease while maintaining cognitive function. Making sure you get enough fats will keep your brain healthy and your mind clear, especially if you also exercise your mind with strategy games like chess or bridge.

Ensuring you have enough of these omega-3 fats in your system can help reduce internal inflammation, which can lead to heart disease and degenerative autoimmune diseases like rheumatoid arthritis. The anti-inflammatory effects also help with exercise recovery, so you can continue your fitness routine without soreness and loss of range of motion.

Omega-3 fats like DHA can also improve eye health. While we don't mainly associate healthy fats with better eyesight, studies have shown that daily supplementation with 600 mg of DHA and 900 mg of EPA improved eye discomfort for those who wear contact lenses and 500 mg of DHA and 1,000 mg of EPS daily for three months lessened eye pressure. This is helpful to ward off glaucoma, since eye pressure is a risk factor for that disease.[2][3]

As we get older, our chances of getting cancer increases, so anything we can do to prevent that from happening is far better and easier than trying to treat the disease. Studies show that people who consume higher amounts of Omega-3 fats lowers overall risk of getting cancer.

According to Science Daily, taking enough omega-3 fatty acid supplements to change the balance of oils in the diet could slow a key biological process linked to aging.

✓The Solution

Add Omega-3's to your diet as often as possible. Best food sources include fish like wild salmon, tuna, herring, sardines and mackerel.

The first goal should always be to meet our nutritional requirements through diet, but when this isn't the case, Omega-3 supplements can help. These include krill oil, cod liver oil, algal oil and some other fish and plant oils combinations. Check your local health food store for the purest sources, and try to get a combination of Omega-3s to ensure you get a full spectrum of nutrients.

2   Downie LE, Gad A, Wong CY, Gray JHV, Zeng W, Jackson DC, Vingrys AJ. Modulating Contact Lens Discomfort With Anti-Inflammatory Approaches: A Randomized Controlled Trial. Invest Ophthalmol Vis Sci. 2018 Jul 2;59(8):3755-3766. doi: 10.1167/iovs.18-24758. PMID: 30046817.

3   Downie LE, Vingrys AJ. Oral Omega-3 Supplementation Lowers Intraocular Pressure in Normotensive Adults. Transl Vis Sci Technol. 2018 May 1;7(3):1. doi: 10.1167/tvst.7.3.1. PMID: 29736322; PMCID: PMC5931260.

Omega 3 to 6 Ratio

Healthy fats provide many benefits from head to toe. But getting the right balance between omega-3 and omega-6 is important in order to reduce oxidative stress and preserve telomeres, the tiny parts of DNA that are related to aging.

Omega-3 and omega-6 fats are both a form of polyunsaturated fats that your body cannot manufacture. Since we need them for good health and many body functions, we have to include them in our diet or through supplementation. But it is not enough simply to consume a lot of both and hope for the best, instead these fats must have a balanced ratio.

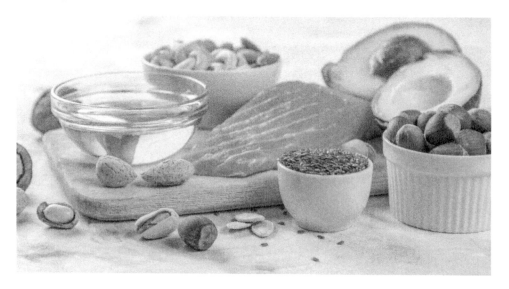

Our modern diets have resulted in an imbalance of omega-3 and omega-6 fatty acids. While the ratio should be 1:1 up to 4:1, of omega-6 and omega-3 respectively, our current average is as high as 20:1. Today, our main source of omega-6 fatty acids come from vegetable oils, which many foods are cooked and fried in. At the same time, we do not get enough omega-3 fatty acids from whole food sources like fatty fish. This is proving to be an imbalanced combination that is aging us faster than our years.

Taking omega-3 fatty acids helps keep the balance of all fatty acids, leading to lowered inflammation, as well. In combination with its effect on telomeres makes it apparent that keeping fats in their proper balance might be a significant nutritional intervention that lowers the risk of many age-related diseases including heart diseases, arthritis, diabetes and Alzheimer's disease.

✓The Solution

Stop cooking with vegetable oils, and instead use ghee, butter or lard, all of which are natural and come with many health benefits. Cooking with unhealthy oils can lead to inflammation, a condition associated with accelerated aging and disease. But cooking with the healthier alternatives like lard provides oleic acid, which supports heart health, and ghee, which is rich in vitamins A, D, K2 and Conjugated Linoleic Acid (CLA), which helps stabilize weight and supports brain and heart health. Butter is also high in vitamin A and CLA, and is best when it is from grass-fed animals.

You can't help getting older, but you don't have to get old.

—**George Burns**

CBD Oil

CBD oil is short for cannabidiol oil and is derived from cannabis of the marijuana plant. While marijuana is associated with smoking pot to get high, CBD oil is an entirely different product. Just like most plant oils, it has many health benefits due to the high amounts of phytochemicals, nine essential amino acids, enzymes, vitamins, minerals, flavonoids and essential fatty acids.

CBD oil contains a host of nutrients including its own B vitamin complex, iron and a host of antioxidants. Along with being highly nutritional, those who advocate CBD oil promote a host of benefits, including it being a good source of iron and complete protein, energy booster and as a pain reliever. But what many people overlook is the potent anti-aging properties and benefits this oil provides.

Relish love in our old age! Aged love is like aged wine; it becomes more satisfying, more refreshing, more valuable, more appreciated and more intoxicating.

—Leo Buscaglia

Pain Relief - The most popular use of this oil is for pain relief, and research does verify that it has anti-inflammatory properties. Inflammation from arthritis causes the pain in the joints, so using anti-inflammatories can provide relief. Researchers agree that CBD oil does have therapeutic potential for pain relief, while at least one study showed it may help with pain from rheumatoid arthritis.[4]

Cell Protection—Cannabidiol, the main component of CBD oil, is one of a group of cannabinoids that works as an antioxidant and helps with

---

4   Malfait AM, Gallily R, Sumariwalla PF, et al. The nonpsychoactive cannabis constituent cannabidiol is an oral anti-arthritic therapeutic in murine collagen-induced arthritis. Proc Natl Acad Sci U S A. 2000;97(17):9561-9566. doi:10.1073/pnas.160105897

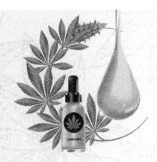

HEALTH BENEFITS OF
CBD OIL

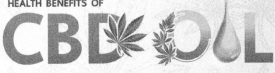

EYES
Compounds found in CBD feature neuro protection and vasodilation properties which furture assist in the conservation and treatment of glaucoma

BRAIN
Anti-Anxiety,Anti-Depressant, Antioxidant, Neuroprotective

BONE STRUCTURE
CBD works by improving bone density and reducing the occurence of bone diseases. it strengths the collagen "bridge" that forms at the site of the break which then hardens with the new bone

HEART
Anti-Inflammatory, Atherosclerosis, and Anti-Ischemic

ASTHMA
CBD has potent immunosuppressive and anti-inflammatory properties

STOMACH
Antiemetic, Appetite Control

INTESTINGS
Cannabidiol reduces intestine inflammation through the control of the neuroimmune system

SPINAL CORD INJURY
Studies have not only demonstrated CBD's pain-killing properties, but also its ability to reduce spasms and improve motor function in SCI patientsv

CANCER
Cannabinoids may have benefits in the treatment of cancer-related side effects

WELL BEING
Helps to relax and to caim body and mind

Relish love in our old age!
Aged love is like aged wine;
it becomes more satisfying,
more refreshing, more
valuable, more appreciated
and more intoxicating.

—Leo Buscaglia

tissue repair and immune protection.[5] We all have natural cannabinoids that attach to cannabinoid receptors, but in this day and age where we come into contact with harmful pathogens and free radicals all day, ever day, providing antioxidants can ensure we do not go into a state of oxidative stress.

Brain Health—Our brains have the ability to change and adapt throughout our lives. The process known as neuro-plasticity keeps our brains young, helps us learn, create memories and even colors the way we see the world. In other words, if we see the world as sad and awful, our thought processes will follow neural pathways that seek out what is sad and awful. On the other hand, if we change our thinking to look for the good in things, our thought patterns will change as the brain creates new pathways for our thoughts to follow. The result of a change in thinking such as this can help you see opportunities that you may have overlooked before, and to see beauty where you once saw only dismay.

This is important for the aging process because of afflictions like depression, forgetfulness, and anxiety. Mature people are more susceptible to Alzheimer's disease and dementia, so we need to do everything we can to preserve and improve brain health. Interestingly, a lack of brain neuroplasticity is linked to the above brain health issues.

Recent studies are showing that cannabinoids increase something called neurotrophic factor (BDNF), which protects brain cells while promot-

---

5   Chen Y, Buck J. Cannabinoids protect cells from oxidative cell death: a receptor-independent mechanism. J Pharmacol Exp Ther. 2000 Jun;293(3):807-12. PMID: 10869379.

ing new cells. This process may help slow down the decline of cognitive functions associated with aging.

When CBD oil is used, it activates our brain's internal cannabinoid system, which helps reduce inflammation of the brain. Triggering this system improves the brain's capacity to remove damaged cells and improve brain cell efficiency, which can potentially ward off Alzheimer's disease.

At least one study showed that CBD induces beneficial plastic changes in the brain, much like clinical antidepressants and antipsychotics. It is also believed that treatment with CBD oil may help alleviate cognitive symptoms associated with neurodegeneration, or aging.[6]

Heart Health—CBD oil helped lower the blood pressure of men during stress tests in one study and is believed to benefits the heart and circulatory system because of this.[7]

Skin Health—Because CBD has great nutritional value and is a rich source of antioxidants, it has a beneficial impact on our skin, as well. Remember that antioxidants combat free radicals that can cause premature aging, which can result in healthier skin. It can also help the skin repair itself, thanks to the effects of the healthy essential fats found in the oil.

✓ The Solution

To get the most anti-aging benefits from CBD oil, find a reputable company and follow the daily recommendations for dosage. Do not worry about getting high or feeling different, because CBD oil does not contain THC, which is the chemical responsible for the feelings of euphoria.

---

6   Campos AC, Fogaça MV, Scarante FF, Joca SRL, Sales AJ, Gomes FV, Sonego AB, Rodrigues NS, Galve-Roperh I, Guimarães FS. Plastic and Neuroprotective Mechanisms Involved in the Therapeutic Effects of Cannabidiol in Psychiatric Disorders. Front Pharmacol. 2017 May 23;8:269. doi: 10.3389/fphar.2017.00269. PMID: 28588483; PMCID: PMC5441138.

7   Jadoon KA, Tan GD, O'Sullivan SE. A single dose of cannabidiol reduces blood pressure in healthy volunteers in a randomized crossover study. JCI Insight. 2017;2(12):e93760. Published 2017 Jun 15. doi:10.1172/jci.insight.93760

Research indicates that CBD is a powerful antioxidant that helps slow down the process of collagen loss as you age. Ultimately, this could help prevent wrinkles and maintain a firm and youthful skin appearance.

CBD oil will come in different potencies, with products that contain more active ingredients costing considerably more. A number that's often in larger print will list the amount of CBD in milligrams for the entire product, not the serving size or dose. On the label, look for the milligrams per milliliter (mg/mL) instead. This is what actually determines the product's concentration of CBD. Potencies can range from 100mg to upwards of 5,000mg for a single 30 ML (1 oz) bottle. The optimal dose and potency will be different for everyone, depending on your needs and health issues you're looking to resolve.

Some anti-aging creams contain CBD oil for topical use. However, some advocates prefer to use their favorite anti-aging creams or body lotions and add the CBD oil to that, which is also perfectly fine.

Medicinal mushrooms

Medicinal mushrooms have been used for thousands of years in traditional remedies. Reishi mushrooms were once called the mushrooms of immortality, and they are used to this day all over the world for promoting health and longevity. Reishi mushrooms are also known to reduce the risk of age-related diseases that can cut life short.

Reishi mushrooms have been traditionally used to cure infections and to boost the immune system. More recently, research is uncovering the anti-cancer properties of this mushroom, and scientists are learning more and hope to develop cancer therapeutics from them.[8]

But reishi mushrooms also have aesthetic value, especially for mature skin. They are deeply hydrating thanks to the polysaccharides, and can help reinforce the moisture barrier so skin retains its softness. It helps reduce inflammation, which can calm skin redness, and the numerous antioxidants provide natural protection from the sun and fight free radicals that cause premature aging.

Chaga mushrooms are similar to reishi in that they have been used in traditional remedies, and it even has a nickname of "black gold." This mushroom species is packed with antioxidants, can lower blood sugar and has been shown to destroy certain cancer cells.

These lesser known mushrooms can help detoxify your blood and can balance your immune system. A balanced immune system is less likely to trigger allergies or develop an autoimmune disease like rheumatoid arthritis. These mushrooms are also high in Betulinic acid, which is known to kill cancer cells while helping skin regenerate itself. And speaking of skin, chaga mushrooms are a great source of melatonin, which can help you get a good night's rest. Between these and reishi mushrooms, you can also build natural sun protection, so you are more protected while also getting your daily dose of vitamin K.

Shiitake mushrooms are used to brighten the skin, and fade sunspots and acne scars. Its anti-inflammatory properties help improve vitality and also encourage faster skin renewal and skin elasticity.

8   Patel S, Goyal A. Recent developments in mushrooms as anti-cancer therapeutics: a review. 3 Biotech. 2012;2(1):1-15. doi:10.1007/s13205-011-0036-2

✓ The Solution

Both reishi and chaga mushrooms can be taken in capsule form, powder form or as a tea. Chaga mushrooms are mainly taken as tea, but never eaten raw because they're hard and not so flavorful. Reishi mushrooms can be eaten fresh or taken as a supplement or extract. When used daily, most consumers prefer supplements because it is simply easier. I believe it is always best to change how you take them from time to time, to keep your body stimulated and happy.

More about Medicinal Mushrooms in my video:

> Channel: The Aging Games
> 5 Natural Ways to Boost Your Immune System - How to Supercharge your Immunity!

Magnesium

Magnesium is a mineral involved in over 300 enzyme reactions and found mostly in the bones, with high concentrations also in the brain and heart. Magnesium deficiencies are dangerous and can lead to many health issues like heart and immune problems. Here are just some benefits:

Nerve Function - Our bodies need magnesium to help convert food into energy, form new proteins, and for a healthy nervous system. When our nervous system is balanced and healthy, nerves remain calm without convulsions or shaking and less prone to seizures. It also means we have more control over our muscles, with both contraction and relaxation, so we experience less cramping and pain.

Heart Health—Low magnesium levels are a risk factor for heart disease and are linked to arterial plaque build-up, hardening of the arteries and high blood pressure. But healthy magnesium levels work with calcium to ensure heart cells and muscle fibers relax after the heartbeat. For some people, magnesium can help with heart palpitations. It is also a key mineral that helps regulate blood pressure.

Blood Sugar Levels—Low magnesium levels are linked to insulin resistance, which is a risk factor for diabetes. Magnesium is responsible for numerous bodily functions, including the regulating of blood sugar. Adequate magnesium intake can help regulate blood sugar to avoid complications that can lead to diabetes.

Better Sleep—As mentioned above, magnesium helps with nerve function and muscle relaxation. In particular, it activates the parasympathetic nervous system, which helps your body relax for the sleep cycle. In addition, it has an effect on something called GABA receptors in the brain, which helps quiet nerves.

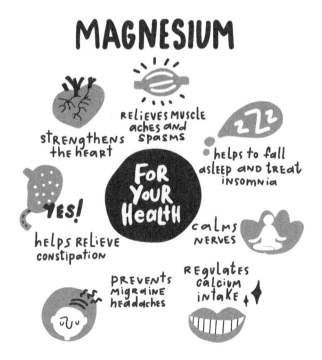

MAGNESIUM

strengthens the heart

RELIEVES MUSCLE aches and spasms

helps to fall asleep and treat insomnia

FOR YOUR Health

YES!

helps RELIEVE constipation

calms NERVES

PREVENTS migraine headaches

REgulates calcium intaKE

Arguably, the most crucial mineral that coffee depletes is magnesium. So in order to maintain healthy magnesium levels, make sure you cut back on caffeinated beverages.

✓ The Solution

Women need about 320 mg of magnesium while men need about 420 mg. According to the National Institutes of Health, most people don't get enough, but you can if you focus on your nutritional needs. Foods that are rich in magnesium include the following:

- Nuts

- Oily Fish

- Yogurt

- Cheese

You can also use a magnesium supplement, but be careful because it can also act as a laxative if you take too much. You can also try a magnesium spray topically to help you sleep at night.

Healthy Microbiome

The microbiome is also called the gut microbiome and is an internal environment that lives inside our digestive tracts. It is filled with trillions of microflora, bacteria and other pathogens that work in harmony to keep hormones balanced and the immune system working. It is also connected with the brain and is the dominant place where the feel-good hormone serotonin is made. And it needs to remain balanced to keep our digestion intact and our entire bodies healthy.

SYMPTOMS OF DYSBIOSIS

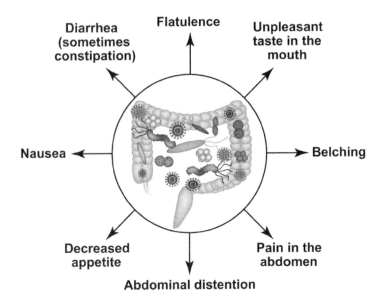

Keeping a balanced microbiome may not be as easy as it seems. It can get thrown off with medication use, too much sugar, overuse of alcohol, and a poor diet. But keeping it healthy has numerous anti-aging effects including:

- Stronger immunity
- Fat metabolism regulation
- Enhanced antioxidant activity
- Reduced internal inflammation

- Prevention of insulin resistance
- Prevention of atherosclerosis
- Prevention of type 2 diabetes
- Prevention of Parkinson's disease

As we get older, our microbiome diversity naturally declines, especially when we reach 60 years of age. At this point, opportunistic bacteria take advantage of the lack of beneficial bacteria, which can make it easier to get infections and chronic diseases. So how do we maintain healthy homeostasis of microbiome as we age?

An unbalanced microbiome can lead to a leaky gut, causing inflammation in the body and dramatically speeding up the aging process.

✓ The Solution

Diet is our main tool to maintain a healthy digestive tract and microbiome. Remove junk and highly processed foods and replace them with healthy, whole foods that are less processed. Remove unhealthy trans fats (like margarine), grains and sugar from your diet and include more meat, seafood and animal fats. Also include foods that promote beneficial bacteria and other healthy pathogens like:

- Fresh sauerkraut
- Kimchi
- Kefir
- Natural yogurt
- Sourdough bread (if you must eat bread)
- Olive oil
- Kombucha in limited amounts
- Ginger

Stress is also a culprit that can sabotage gut health. Try relaxing meditation for 10-15 minutes each day, and be sure to get enough sleep through the night.

Check out my Guided Meditation Video for Stress and Anxiety:

Channel: The Aging Games
Guided Meditation for letting go of Stress and Anxiety

And my Guided Meditation for Deep Sleep:

Channel: The Aging Games
Guided Meditation for Sleep | Natural Relaxing way to
Fight Insomnia

Castor Oil

Castor oil (also known as Palm of Christ) is a very versatile oil that has been used for centuries to promote health and beauty and is especially beneficial to nourish the hair, skin and liver.

The oil comes from the castor bean, which contains a healthy fatty acid called ricinoleic acid, which fights inflammation and is said to promote hair growth. The unsaturated fatty acids can feed the hair follicles at the source and your scalp can take advantage of the omega-6 and omega-9s along with vitamin E, which is considered a hair elixir combination. Also, true castor oil stimulates blood vessel dilation, so when applied topically, blood vessels have an increased capacity to feed nutrient and oxygen rich blood to the hair follicles and hair root.

Thick lashes and eyebrows can also result from topically applied castor oil. And while there may not be much scientific research, the internet is full of before and after photos of advocates who use the remedy at home and prove it does have a positive effect. Please check out my own experience with castor oil in this video:

Channel: The Aging Games
Castor Oil for Hair Growth | Grow long Eyelashes and
thick Eyebrows

If you have never used castor oil before, try a skin spot allergy test before use.

✓The Solution

Hair: Advocates of castor oil for hair growth suggest massaging just a few drops of cold-pressed castor oil onto your scalp and leave it for at least two hours before you wash it out. You can also leave it on overnight. If you like, add a few drops down the hair shafts, as well to get rid of frizziness or split ends.

Eyebrows and Lashes: At bedtime, be sure to remove all makeup from your face, lashes and brows and remove contacts if you wear them. Dip a cotton swab into the cold-pressed castor oil and apply it to the top of your lash line, being careful to avoid dripping into the eye. Apply to your eyebrows in the same way. Cleanse your eyelashes and brows in the morning with makeup remover.

Castor Oil Packs

In this section, we will explore castor oil for helping do detoxify the liver. Castor oil is an ancient remedy for helping clear the liver of waste. Today, we need to help our livers more than ever before thanks to the use of numerous chemicals and pesticides in our food, beverages and even water. Many of us are familiar with ingesting healthy oils, but this is another topical use of castor oil. Applied 2-3 times per week, the benefits will include improved circulation, hormonal support, pain relief and liver detoxification.

In this method, you add castor oil to a cloth and allow it to seep into your skin, using heat. The practice has been taught in many schools of alternative and traditional medicines and is still used to this day as it is easy, relaxing and effective. It has been used as a wound healer, but it also seems to increase T-11 immune cells, which eliminate viruses, bacteria and even cancer cells. Some believe the topical application of castor oil with heat activates lymphocytes in the skin, leading to the overall immune stimulating reaction.

✓The Solution

- Purchase pure castor oil and castor oil packing material or cloth from your local health store. (Many stores place these next to each other to make it easy for the customer to find.) It can also be purchased online.

- Lie in a comfortable place where you will enjoy resting for about an hour, with a heating pad.

- Pour 2 to 4 tablespoons of castor oil onto the cloth and place it on the liver area of your body, which is your right side, back, lower part of the ribcage.

- Cover with plastic to avoid leaking onto your sofa or bed.

- Place a heating pad on medium or low over the pack and rest.

- Relax from 40 minutes up to 1 ½ hours, however long you are comfortable.

- Try doing this at least 2-3 times a week.

- Some people prefer to follow with a water enema the next day.

This is a very gentle liver detox that is highly tolerable and effective.

Liver Flush

This liver flush is a little more aggressive than the above one, and is based on the works of Ayurvedic practitioner, Andreas Moritz. It is one of the most popular and effective ways to help your body remove gallstones and is an effective tool to improve your health at any age.

One thing Andreas Moritz learned was that it seemed every patient suffering from chronic illness also had a large number of gallstones. Normally thought to be located in the gallbladder, mainstream medicine will wait until one blocks the bile ducts, then will either try to remove it surgically or remove your entire gallbladder.

Getting old is a fascination thing. The older you get, the older you want to get.

—**Keith Richards**

Moritz found that stones can also form in the liver, where they may be called bile stones, but they can cause the same problems. The stones are made of cholesterol, calcium salts, bile and minerals. They may be tiny like sand or as large as a pebble, hard or soft, and one liver can contain up to 6,000 stones before one feels the effect! Needless to say, it may be healthier to try to help your body eliminate them before they begin to suffocate your organs.

✓ The Solution

Prepare for your liver flush by consuming a healthy diet, 4 to 6 glasses of fresh water throughout the day and 32 ounces of organic, unfiltered apple juice, 9 ounces of sour cherry juice or malic acid capsules if you prefer not to do the juices. Do this every day for five days.

Day 6:

1. On day six, drink either the apple juice or sour cherry juice only while abstaining from food (fasting).

2. Cleanse: Mix 2 Tablespoons of Epsom salt with 12 ounces of filtered water and drink 6 ounces at 6pm and 6 ounces at 8pm.

3. At 10pm, drink 4 ounces of olive oil mixed with 6 ounces of grapefruit juice or 4 ounces of pure lemon juice. (Some people add stevia to make it more palatable.)

4. It is imperative to go to bed now and lie flat on your back with your head on a pillow. Lie still for at least 20 minutes. Try to sleep for the night.

Day 7:

1. At 6am drink 1 Tablespoon of Epsom salt with 1 cup of water (add lemon juice and/or stevia if needed)

2. 8am drink 1 Tablespoon of Epsom salt with 1 cup of water, again

3. Lie down again for at least 20 minutes.

You should eventually have bowel movements that may begin at the end of day 6, the morning of day 7 or in between.

Doing this liver flush regularly will penetrate deeper and deeper into the liver to eliminate bile stones. You will feel younger, fresher, with more energy with each flush. It is also very helpful for weight loss, as a toxic liver will be

Blotchy skin, acne, wrinkles, and dark circles can affect our confidence in a very profound way. People don't realize that unsightly skin issues may actually be caused by the accumulation of toxins in the liver.

interfering with any weight loss efforts. You may also see liver spots disappear from the hands and face.

Please check with your medical provider before embarking on a liver flush, especially if you have any underlying health conditions.

Activate AMPK Enzyme

Adenosine monophosphate activated protein kinase (AMPK) is an important enzyme that is crucial for energy metabolism. And not only does it keep our metabolism revved, but it can help your body burn more fat, build muscle, help reduce insulin resistance and decrease inflammation, all of which help slow down the aging process.

Getting old is a fascination thing. The older you get, the older you want to get.

—Keith Richards

While it sounds like a miracle pill, AMPK is present in all of our cells. Studies show that not only does it have the above health benefits, but it can help reverse diabetes, improve heart health, and extend our life span. But, since it isn't a pill, how do we take advantage of this enzyme? Due to its importance, the majority of the discussion is in the solution.

✓ The Solution

- **Do Not Overeat** - This natural enzyme decreases with age, as most do, which is why taking care of yourself is imperative to allow the body to remain healthy for as long as possible. Overeating is a practice that can overload the body, causing cell maintenance functions to decrease or stop, altogether. Unfortunately, this also seems to lessen the activation and activity of AMPK, because the cells cannot metabolize energy if it is always in the process of digestion. Therefore, the practice of abstaining from overeating is the beginning of activating this enzyme.

- **Exercise**—High intensity exercise activates AMPK in skeletal muscle, as it helps repair damage resulting from the workout.

- **Low Carbs**— High carbohydrate intake increases insulin, resulting in high blood sugar. Eventually, this decreases our overall AMPK levels. Sticking to a low carbohydrate diet can help overcome this.

- **Healthy Fats**—Omega-3 fats help reduce inflammation, which has a direct effect on AMPK activity. It seems that chronic internal inflammation inhibits this enzyme, while omega-3 fatty acids increase a hormone called adiponectin, which activates AMPK.

Supplements that can help AMPK activation:

- *Resveratrol*
- *Alpha Lipoic Acid*
- *Gynostemma*
- *Quercetin*

Telomeres and DNA Health

Telomeres are the most studied link to aging in the human body. Telomeres are protein structures at the end of each strand of DNA. Cells divide during their lifetime, as part of our normal cell processes. Each time a cell divides, telomeres become shorter, until it reaches a critical limit, and the cell will no longer divide, marking the end of the cell's lifespan. Scientists associate with length of one's telomeres to determine lifespan.

It may seem like something that is completely beyond our control, but there are things we can do to protect our telomeres and DNA. A study with the Preventive Medicine Research Institute found that our telomeres are not set in stone and may be "lengthened" through lifestyle changes. In the study, some men were given lifestyle changes that included stress management, exercise, diet and social support, while a control group had no change. The telomeres of the control group shortened during the 5-year study while telomeres and telomerase enzyme activity of the men who incorporated lifestyle changes had increased.[9]

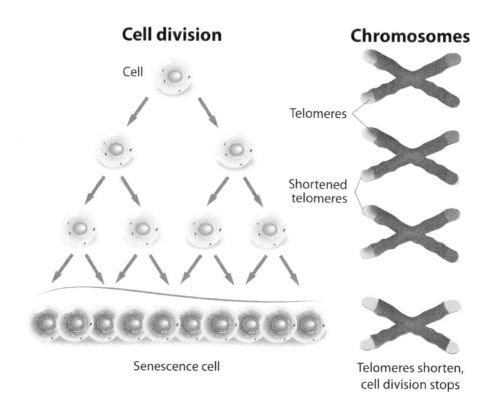

Cell division

Cell

Senescence cell

Chromosomes

Telomeres

Shortened telomeres

Telomeres shorten, cell division stops

9   Ornish D, Lin J, Chan JM, Epel E, Kemp C, Weidner G, Marlin R, Frenda SJ, Magbanua MJM, Daubenmier J, Estay I, Hills NK, Chainani-Wu N, Carroll PR, Blackburn EH. Effect of comprehensive lifestyle changes on telomerase activity and telomere length in men with biopsy-proven low-risk prostate cancer: 5-year follow-up of a descriptive pilot study. Lancet Oncol. 2013 Oct;14(11):1112-1120. doi: 10.1016/S1470-2045(13)70366-8. Epub 2013 Sep 17. PMID: 24051140.

✓The Solution

According to the above, the solution for maintaining healthy DNA includes the following:

- Exercise regularly

- Maintain a healthy weight

- Incorporate a healthy diet based on animal proteins and healthy fats

Extra Telomere Points

- Include foods that are associated with increased lifespan and longer telomeres such as berries, mushrooms and foods high in Omega-3 such as cold water fish

- Incorporate supplements that are also associated with healthy DNA like omega-3 fatty acids, N-acetyle-cysteine (NAC) to support glutathione, an internal antioxidant, vitamin D and astragalus. Innovative supplement companies offer supplements that incorporate several healthy nutrients that may help lengthen or preserve telomeres.

> *Telomeres shorten each time a cell copies itself. Eventually, telomeres get too short to do their job, causing our cells to age and stop functioning adequately. Therefore, telomeres act as the aging clock in every cell.*

In the end, it's not the years in your life that count. It's the life in your years.

—Abraham Lincoln

CHAPTER 5

Home Therapies & Exercise

Home therapies are grouped with exercise because, like exercise, they involve full-body activities. Some people consider certain types of exercise to be home therapies, while some home therapies are so powerful some health practitioners equate them to exercise. These are all healthy practices that can have a wonderfully beneficial impact on our lives and health.

Infrared Sauna

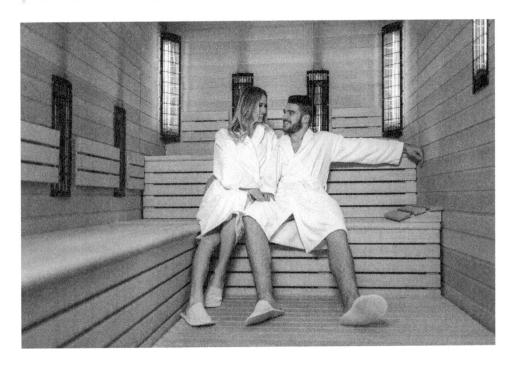

Infrared saunas are used by many as part of a healthy lifestyle to help the body detoxify, increase circulation, and help muscle recovery, especially after exercise. Each of these is directly related to the aging process and how age is biologically expressed through our bodies. Here are some benefits:

Improved Skin—Researchers of one study decided to follow through and see why Infrared heat was consistently used for aesthetic and health

Infrared saunas for skin care are one of the top natural anti-aging tools you can find. Infrared waves penetrate deep into the skin to increase circulation, detoxify, improve complexion, and reduce wrinkles.

purposes. They found that skin exposed to infrared heat increased the production of elastin and collagen, and the benefits continued with regular use. After 6 months of treatment, subjects reported improvements in skin texture, tone and smoothness.[1]

Less Stress—Chronic stress can cause fatigue, lead to a poor diet, can negatively impact the brain and is even linked to many diseases that are also common to aging. But learning to cope with stress can help us in every aspect of aging from skin quality to living without disease. Practicing stress management in an infrared sauna can be very effective, as it can also lower blood pressure during the session.

Improve Circulation—The heat from an infrared sauna increases circulation while you relax. This allows your blood to carry more oxygen and nutrients throughout your body, which can result in better health, improved skin quality and some believe lengthened telomeres, since the circulatory effect is similar to exercise.

✓ The Solution

Infrared saunas can be found in spas or bought online for home use. Blankets and other home devices sell for as little as $200, with full home saunas costing up to $4,000 and more. These are some of the best practices for infrared sauna use:

• Be sure to drink plenty of water before and after

1   Lee JH, Roh MR, Lee KH. Effects of infrared radiation on skin photo-aging and pigmentation. Yonsei Med J. 2006;47(4):485-490. doi:10.3349/ymj.2006.47.4.485

- Don't wear clothing inside the sauna

- Eat a healthy diet to support your body's detoxing processes

- Begin with 10 minutes and slowly work your way up

- Practice mindfulness techniques like relaxation or self-hypnosis to get the most out of your session.

Red Light Therapy

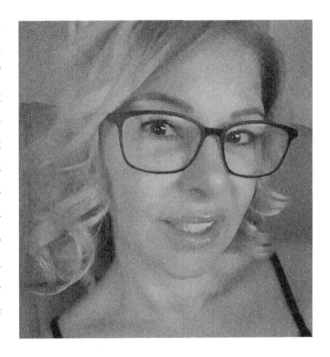

Red light therapy (RLT) is similar to Infrared Light, except it's visible to the human eye. RLT is also known as low-power light therapy and low-level laser therapy (LLLT), and is a treatment that exposes the body and cells to low wavelength red light. Mitochondria, which are the powerhouses of our cells, can absorb the light particles and use them to produce more adenosine triphosphate (ATP), a molecule that turns food into fuel.

A review of studies shows that RLT has a wide range of applications and can stimulate skin rejuvenation, help reduce inflammation and stimulate healing, all things that can help slow the aging process. Within this review, it is pointed out that LLLT (same as RLT) is effective at improving wrinkles and tightening the skin.[2] But that's not all RLT can do.

---

2   Avci P, Gupta A, Sadasivam M, et al. Low-level laser (light) therapy (LLLT) in skin: stimulating, healing, restoring. Semin Cutan Med Surg. 2013;32(1):41-52.

Another review of several studies found that LLLT is an effective treatment for healing skin wounds.[3] This is important for the aging process, because as we mature the immune system slows down, leading to slower wound healing and skin rejuvenation. Accelerating the healing process not only helps our skin, but could indicate that RLT has a beneficial impact on our entire immune system.

> Relish love in our old age! Aged love is like aged wine; it becomes more satisfying, more refreshing, more valuable, more appreciated and more intoxicating.
>
> **—Leo Buscaglia**

Aside from the studies, there is enough anecdotal evidence that RLT has many additional benefits. Dermatologists around the world use it as a treatment to reduce wrinkles and tighten skin, and millions of people undergo the treatment every year. Many plastic surgeons now offer RLT for their patients for quicker recovery after any type of surgery. In addition, tens of thousands of RLT devices are sold for home use with raving reviews. Traditionally, if a treatment didn't work or had too many side effects, it would eventually fade out, so RLT is withstanding the test of time.

In a small study, subjects with dementia underwent RLT for 12 weeks. The result was improved sleep, improved mood (those with dementia often experience anger), and had better memory recollection. And yet another small study found that RLT helped those with androgenetic alopecia (a disorder that causes hair loss) helped subjects grow thicker hair, compared to a placebo group that used a fake RLT device. Some spas and treatment centers use red light therapy for targeted weight loss, be-

---

3   Chaves ME, Araújo AR, Piancastelli AC, Pinotti M. Effects of low-power light therapy on wound healing: LASER x LED. An Bras Dermatol. 2014;89(4):616-623. doi:10.1590/abd1806-4841.20142519

cause some studies show that it promotes fat cell apoptosis, or fat cell death.

Each of these smaller studies is criticized because they are small, but it may be because the technology is just now being brought into the spotlight with the many treatments that it is being used for. Fortunately, RLT is considered effective and safe for just about anyone, including pets.

Please check out my video about Red Light Therapy for more info:

Channel: The Aging Games
Can Red Light Therapy Help you Reverse Aging?

√ The Solution

Red light therapy sessions are available at spas around the world. Some dermatologists offer a facial or body treatment for wrinkles, while others offer targeting areas of the body to promote fat loss. Gyms, spas, and tanning salons also offer RLT for various purposes and prices. The cost can range from as low as $45 per session to hundreds of dollars per session, with most people requiring multiple treatments.

Many health professionals promote the use of home devices for RLT. Devices range from helmets that provide red lights to wear for stimulation of hair growth, boxes of red lights that are directed at you as you rest and handheld wands for facial treatments. Another easy way to incorporate red light therapy at home is to purchase red light lamps to place around your home, so you can simply sit

Count your age by friends, not years. Count your life by smiles, not tears.

—**John Lennon**

Infrared light therapy is very useful in helping to reduce bruising and swelling after surgery, particularly when it is used in the first few days after surgery. It can speed the healing process and help restore the tissues that have been subjected to some trauma from surgery.

under them at your convenience. RLT can be done every day, but just like anything else, not excessively.

Epsom Salt Baths

Epsom salt baths are an easy and relaxing way to help your body detoxify. It is traditionally used for pain relief, especially for post-workout soreness. But, aside from relaxing in a tub after a workout, how is adding Epsom salt to your bath work as an anti-aging hack?

Epsom salt is really magnesium sulfate, which is a chemical compound that includes magnesium, oxygen and sulfur. In spite of its name, it is not the same as table salt, and when dissolved it releases magnesium and sulfate ions. Some chiropractors claim that during a warm, Epsom salt bath, these ions are absorbed into the pads of the intervertebral discs, which helps them balance, thus relaxing the spine in a natural manner.

We know that magnesium is an important mineral necessary for hundreds of enzyme reactions throughout the body. These enzyme reactions help the body heal and function. And while we don't have scientific evidence that this magnesium is absorbed through the skin, we must consider that the skin is a porous organ that absorbs toxic ingredients from topical creams, pollutants and chemicals from the workplace and even from air pollution. If the skin does this, then we can deduce that the skin also has the ability to absorb healthy minerals like magnesium from Epsom salt.

✓ The Solution

1. Drink some fresh, spring water before your bath. If you are on a full body cleanse or detox, taking an Epsom salt bath during some or all of the days can support the process.

2. Add about 2 cups of Epsom salt to your bath. Make the water as warm as you can handle without burning or becoming overly fatigued and relax in the water for at least 15 minutes.

3. To make the bath more relaxing and beneficial, add a few drops of pure essential oils like lavender to promote healing and relaxation, or rose oil for beautiful skin.

4. If your heartbeat becomes rapid or overly strong, the water may have been too hot or you may have been in too long, so it is time to get out.

Epsom salt helps reduce the appearance of wrinkles on the face and body, by making the skin softer and more hydrated. Although it may not be as effective for deeper wrinkles, it helps with the fine lines that form around the eyes and mouth.

Those who love deeply never grow old; they may die of old age, but they die young.

—Ben Franklin

Cold Therapy

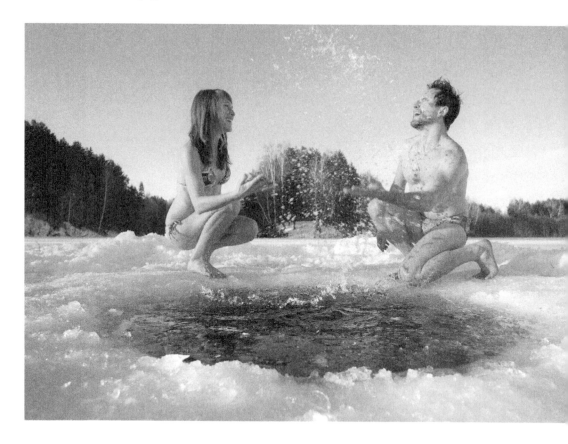

Cold therapy is also called cryotherapy or cold thermogenesis and is commonly used to treat pain. But it can be used to reduce inflammation and swelling, stimulate your immune system, and even to support fat loss and weight control. For anti-aging, the benefits include collagen boosting, increased metabolism and cellulite reduction.

Cold water therapy has been used by Native Americans for creating energy, vitality, and health. The Ancient Greeks used alternating heat and cold therapy for healing and improved circulation. And today, aesthetic practitioners and dermatologists use a form of cold therapy to "freeze" off fat and to tone the skin.

Cold therapy is used by many today as a therapy to tighten the skin through vasodilation, which brings more oxygen and nutrients to the skin. Many experts claim it can also reduce puffiness and dark circles under the eyes.

Cryotherapy is another term for cold therapy, but is more often associated

I am appalled that the term we use to talk about aging is 'anti.' Aging is as natural as a baby's softness and scent. Aging is human evolution in its pure form.

—**Jamie Lee Curtis**

with expensive treatments that are performed in spas. It may be used as I mentioned above, for targeted tightening or fat loss, while some facilities offer sessions in a box much like an infrared sauna where one stands and freezes for about three minutes.

These treatments may be trending; however, you can use cold therapy at home yourself, and experience the benefits like increased metabolism, which needs support as we get older. Many advocates of cold therapy report increased energy, especially when used at the beginning of the day. It also seems to help relieve pain and other symptoms from certain autoimmune diseases. And some who follow a method using cold therapy along with breathing exercises are able to reduce the amount of pain medications they take, lessen symptoms of arthritis and improve their overall immunity.[4]

Lastly, exposure to cold temperatures activates the sympathetic nervous system while increasing endorphins. Because of this, some health prac-

4   Buijze GA, Sierevelt IN, van der Heijden BC, Dijkgraaf MG, Frings-Dresen MH. The Effect of Cold Showering on Health and Work: A Randomized Controlled Trial [published correction appears in PLoS One. 2018 Aug 2;13(8):e0201978]. PLoS One. 2016;11(9):e0161749. Published 2016 Sep 15. doi:10.1371/journal.pone.0161749

titioners have recommended cold shower therapies as a way to combat depression and improve one's overall disposition.

Check out my video for more info:

Channel: The Aging Games
Cold Therapy for Weight Loss Anti-Aging and Better Immunity

✓ The Solution

Cold therapy can be performed at home safely and effectively. But many find cold therapy to be very uncomfortable, especially in cold temperature areas, where a warm bath is comforting and soothing. There is a way to ease yourself into the practice, however.

Begin by taking a shower and alternate the water temperature from warm to cool. Only go as warm or as cool as you can tolerate comfortably. Allow the temperature to remain there for 20-30 seconds before going to the other extreme. You will find that the difference in temperatures may not be that much, at first.

After taking a shower like this two or three times, push yourself by cooling the water a little more, and only for about 10 seconds. After more showers, you will find that you can easily tolerate more extreme temperatures for a longer time. This is mainly because the cold-water part stimulates the entire body, and you will feel more awake and invigorated because of it. Interestingly, those who practice this find they have more energy and less muscle soreness than after a long, hot shower.

As you get used to the colder parts of your shower, try experimenting with a 10-minute-long cold shower with no warm alternates. At this point, you should be able to endure the time and temperature, and thus enjoy the most benefits from cold therapy.

Cold adaptation doesn't take very long and you can help the process along by not overdressing as the temperatures start to drop and also not overheating the house. Sleeping in a cold room is also ideal, very healing and promotes restful sleep. Once you're cold adapted, you can experiment with outdoor swimming in the winter and ice baths in addition to cold showers.

Dunking your face in cold ice water is also a great practice for tightening the skin and getting rid of puffiness and inflammation. You can try dunking your face for 10-15 seconds and repeat three times. Best to do this in the morning.

Wim Hof and Dr. Jack Kruse both have a lot of very useful information on the benefits of cold therapy and Wim Hof also includes a series of breathing exercises to help the process. Please don't dismiss this therapy too quickly as it truly is a life changing hack.

Cold therapy has been reported to improve hormonal response and balancing, almost like a reset of this internal thermostat. The consequence of this leads to reductions in hot flushes during the menopause and therefore less of those embarrassing moments and sleepless nights.

Do not grow old, no matter how long you live. Never cease to stand like curious children before the great mystery into which we were born.

—Albert Einstein

Grounding or Earthing

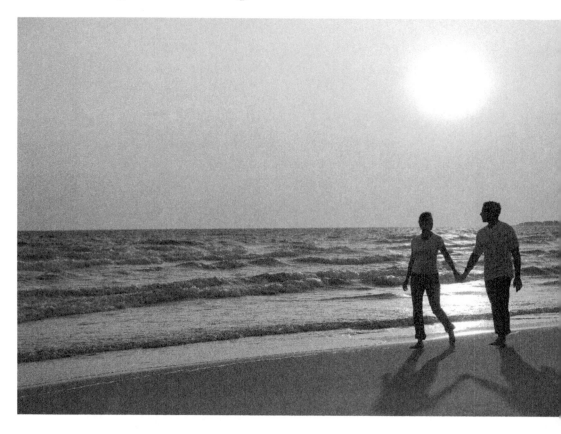

Grounding and earthing are the same thing, which is deliberately bringing direct, physical contact between the earth and the human body. While this might sound a bit like something from a fairy tale, science is beginning to uncover the benefits of the practice including an improvement in the quality of blood so it is less prone to clumping, lowering the risk for heart attacks. Other studies showed it supported the cardiovascular system and improved heart rate variability and had lower risk of arthritis, asthma, sleep apnea and pain reduction.[5]

5   Chevalier G, Sinatra ST, Oschman JL, Sokal K, Sokal P. Earthing: health implications of reconnecting the human body to the Earth's surface electrons. J Environ Public Health. 2012;2012:291541. doi:10.1155/2012/291541

One theory among researchers recognizes the fact that energy and electrical currents run through the entire body, and so connecting with the "vast supply of electrons" on Earth may be the force that promotes physiological changes.[6]

Let's explore some of the benefits.

- Grounding reduces the inflammatory response, reduces pain and even affects white blood cells like lymphocytes, so the immune system works better.

- Thermal imaging cameras can record changes in skin temperatures and show that grounding helps reduce inflammation from injury.

- A "grounded sleep system" consisting of a cotton sheet with carbon threads, connected to a rod inserted into the soil outside improves quality of sleep and fewer aches and pains through the night and upon awakening.

- Earthing seems to cancel out the negative effects of electrical systems around us, including radiation from cell phones.

- Earthing helps reduce stress markers with an overall reduction in tension in grounded subjects.

- Grounding is so powerful a report in the Journal of Environmental Health, researchers exclaimed that this is a missing link in health and should hold the same importance as diet, fresh water, sunshine, exercise and fresh air.[7]

---

6   Chevalier G, Sinatra ST< Oschman JL, Sokal K, Sokal P. Earthing: health implications of reconnecting the human body to the Earth's surface electrons. J Environ Public Health. 2012;2012:291541. doi:10.1155/2012/291541

7   Gaétan Chevalier, Stephen T. Sinatra, James L. Oschman, Karol Sokal, Pawel Sokal, "Earthing: Health Implications of Reconnecting the Human Body to the Earth's Surface Electrons", Journal of Environmental and Public Health, vol. 2012, Article ID 291541, 8 pages, 2012. https://doi.org/10.1155/2012/291541

Grounding to the Earth can decrease hormonal fluctuations, eliminate hot flashes, lift one's mood, and increase the quality of sleep.

√ The Solution

While grounding might sound like a miracle cure, it really is and the best part is, it's very easy to incorporate into anyone's life. Just like diet, exercise and meditation, the benefits are compounded when other healthy lifestyle factors are combined into your daily routine.

• The easiest and most accessible way to incorporate earthing into your health regimen is simply to connect with the earth by sitting, lying, or walking on the earth with direct contact.

• Go for a walk or hike in nature while barefoot

• Swim in the ocean

• Walk on the beach barefoot

• Sleep on the ground with only cotton between you and the ground

• If you have a choice of your indoor environment, cement floors that are not painted or sealed are good conductors and a way to access the earth's energy

• Earthing products allow you to incorporate even more grounding or earthing into your everyday life. These include mattresses, sheets, auto seat pads and sleeping bags as just some tools that can help. There could be some issues with this, and you need to make sure your house is properly grounded.

Inversion Therapy

Inversion therapy is what is sounds like, inverting your body so you are suspended, upside down. This technique is performed with an inversion device that helps you hang upside down, allowing your spine to stretch and release all tension. This takes all the pressure off your back and allows improved blood flow, flow of spinal fluid and a myriad of other benefits that are especially helpful for mature people.

Improved circulation is one of the most effective ways to bring more life-giving oxygen to all areas of your body, as well as increase the transportation of nutrients. The following are more benefits, in detail.

Inversion helps decompress the vertebrae. By relieving pressure on discs, the body can better rehydrate them, reduce nerve pressure and thus help the spine realign itself. Older people have had a lifetime of pressure on their spines, no matter whether we are sitting or standing. This cuts off circulation and fluids that bring essential nutrients. But using inversion therapy daily can help your spine heal.

Inter-vertebrae disc health improves with inversion therapy. Sitting, standing and even lying down all compress the spine and the fluid filled discs in between each vertebra. Over time, compression of these discs can cause us to lose half an inch or more in height. Aside from being shorter, this means the discs are less pliable and provide less cushioning, leading to back pain, loss of motion and even problems

In spite of illness, in spite even of the archenemy sorrow, one can remain alive long past the usual date of disintegration if one is unafraid of change, insatiable in intellectual curiosity, interested in big things, and happy in small ways.

—**Edith Wharton**

with muscles surrounding the spine. Inversion therapy stretches the spine and opens the spaces in between, so the discs expand. During this time, healthy fluid exchange can take place, as the discs renew themselves.

Ease nerve pressure of the spine. When discs shrink and the spine becomes less aligned, surrounding nerves may succumb to pinching and squeezing, causing pressure and pain. The spinal cord is not the boney vertebrae, but a bundle of nerves that are located within it. Compression of the spine and discs often result in pinched nerves, a painful condition that can cause one to become bedridden. But inversion therapy can help lengthen the spine, allowing more room for the spinal cord.

Anti-aging benefits. Most people who invest in inversion tables are looking to eliminate back pain and reduce pressure on their spines. But it actually goes much deeper than this. Inversion therapy is a great way to relax after a busy day, stimulate your internal organs for improved digestion, and improve your posture, sleep and the function of the lymphatic system. All of these will lead to tremendous benefits when it comes to aging. And let's not forget about the part gravity plays in the ageing process. With Inversion Therapy, you can reverse the effects of gravity on your skin and body and see a visible difference while also becoming stronger and more toned all over.

Aging isn't about getting old it's about LIVING… Learning that you can age well, will actually help you to age better… let's start celebrating and living an engaged life, and stop punishing ourselves for not looking a certain way, and instead holding ourselves accountable for actually taking care of ourselves inside first, knowing the results on the exterior will be a shining side effect.

—Cameron Diaz

✓The Solution

Inversion therapy can be performed in a number of ways, and luckily you don't have to be completely upside down.

- An inversion chair is a device that will bring you to an angle that is comfortable and beneficial. Sitting in the chair is preferable for some who are uncomfortable with the foot apparatus used with the inversion table.

- An inversion table is the most widely recognized and popular device. By lying on the table, you can raise your arms above your head until you are upside down.

- Inversion boots are the least expensive option and can be hung from a chin-up bar.

- Yoga poses including headstands, shoulder stands, handstands and the plow pose are forms of inversion therapy without an apparatus.

- An aerial scarf or yoga trapeze requires a tall room and some skill, but may be one of the most creative and enjoyable ways to achieve inversion.

- Check with your doctor if you have medical conditions, as this may increase blood pressure or eye pressure for some people.

Inversion increases circulation, which can support the movement of hormones through the body, reducing mood swings and counteracting any insomnia, as well as reducing stress.

Facial Exercises

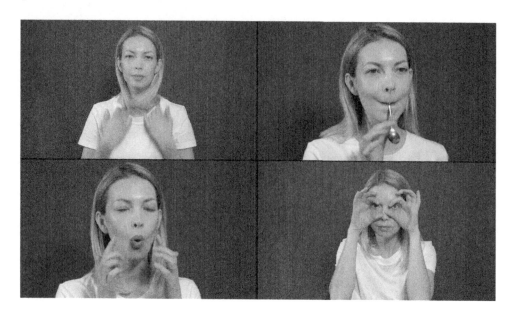

Many people run to the plastic surgeon for Botox and fillers at the earliest signs of sagging skin, but you may be able to ward off the signs of aging by tightening your skin at home. Facial exercise comes in many forms, from daily exercises to face yoga. Each method is based on the premise that holding the shape of the face are muscles, which are prone to sagging, just like any other muscle in your body. And just like other muscles, they can be tightened and strengthened with exercise.

This is yet another field that does not have scientific studies behind it, but most advocates claim they don't need it. Simply try the exercises for a couple weeks and you will see a difference yourself. The exercises are easy to do at home alone or with an inexpensive device. Each area of the face has its own exercise, and you can put together exercise for areas that you feel need improvement.

Facial exercises not only tighten muscles that support face skin, but the increased activity brings more circulation to the skin, resulting in a healthier complexion. Facial yoga is slightly different in that the movements release tension and strain, allowing the face to appear more relaxed and rejuvenated. Facial yoga also results in increased circulation for a healthier complexion.

The face and neck have more than 55 muscles that can be toned. Some exercises feel more like a stretch while some compress. Certain devices make it easy to exercise muscles, which makes is easier to stick with a daily routine. Some critics feel that facial exercises will increase wrinkles, but this is easily combatted by paying attention to how you are moving your face, use the right serums for moisturizing and be sure to keep up a healthy diet so your body has resilience and can continue to manufacture collagen to combat fine lines and wrinkles.

Yawning and opening the mouth as far as possible, then closing it very slowly without letting the teeth touch can help improve the jowls. Repeat 20 times.

✓The Solution

- Find a set routine of facial exercises or put one together for yourself by searching online.

- If you prefer, look for an exercise device

- Moisturize your face and do a light massage from neck to forehead

- Either sit up straight or lie on your back (best position) and perform the facial exercises

- When complete, gently massage each area of your face again for about 10 seconds

- Stop doing intense cardio and running

- Hold devices at eye level. Looking down all day will cause early jowls to form.

- Build more muscle—weight training is so important for strong bones, posture and fat burning

HIIT Your Workout

HIIT stands for High Intensity Interval Training and is one of the quickest ways to burn fat and get into shape. Most HIIT classes held at gyms can be very intense, so it may be best to try this at home yourself first. The benefits are worth it, and most fitness experts agree that you can get in shape with HIIT in a shorter time than with any other exercise programs.

It turns out that HIIT routines are the best fitness regimen to burn fat and reverse the aging process. Most people are familiar with the benefits of exercise for aging, like:

- Stronger bones and improved bone density

- Less muscle wasting, while sculpting lean, strong muscles

- Increased metabolism

- Improved hormonal health

- Improve mental outlook and self-esteem

- Increased energy

- Improved sleep

But HIIT specifically stands out when it comes to anti-aging and fat burning. Check out some details about the benefits:

Protein synthesis is the ability of a muscle to rebuild itself and diminished protein synthesis is a sign of aging. Older muscles have a more difficult time producing protein. But researchers and the Mayo Clinic found that incorporating a HIIT routine enhances protein synthesis, allowing even older people to build or repair muscle.

Mitochondrial activity is the act of producing energy from the cells to our muscles and organs. Regular training with a HIIT routine enhances this process. In fact, one study showed that -incorporating a 25-minute HIIT routine five days per week, with three days of cycling and two days of walking for 12 weeks resulted in improved mitochondrial activity for both young and mature people. However, while the age group of 18 to 30 had a 49% improvement, those aged 65 to 80 years experienced a 69% improvement in mitochondrial activity in the same amount of time!

Muscle mass also improved and increased for both groups, as well as improved aerobic capacity. These benefits are also linked to the improvement of mitochondrial activity and maintaining fitness on a cellular level is proving to play a role in longevity.

Telomeres lengthened in one study. As we discussed earlier, telomere length is directly related to our health and biological age. This part of the DNA shortens as cells die and the ability to regenerate become less as we age. But in this study, 8 weeks of HIIT sessions performed just 3 times a week for young men that were not athletes re-

Mitochondria contribute to specific aspects of the aging process including cellular senescence, chronic inflammation and the age-dependent decline in stem cell activity.

sulted in what researchers called a significant increase in telomere length and telomerase activity.[8]

✓ The Solution

HIIT is performed by exercising in intervals; use "all-out" exertion alternated with active rest. Here is a sample routine for those who walk or jog:

- Warm up for 5 minutes

- Sprint for 20 seconds

- Walk for 90 seconds

- Repeat 5 times

- Walk slowly for 5 minutes to cool down

- Walking and sprinting can be replaced with walking and jogging, interval cycling, swimming and even boxing

While HIIT sounds like an enticing go-to exercise, for the best effects aim for two to three days a week, and do strength training for one or two days each week. Some people use HIIT with weights or kettlebell workouts, which can be found online.

Yoga, Stretching and Thai Chi

These exercises are grouped together as they are very similar. Each involves slow, deliberate movements. The poses help stretch and open up muscles, tendons and ligaments while improving blood flow into these same areas. When performed properly, they can also help open up your internal organs, allowing for more oxygen and nourishment to reach

---

8   Noorimofrad, Saeedreza & Ebrahim, Khosrow. (2018). The effect of high intensity interval training on telomere length and telomerase activity in non-athlete young men. Journal of Basic Research in Medical Sciences. 5. 1-7. 10.29252/jbrms.5.2.1.

them. As we age, this is extremely important, for a nourished and well oxygenated organ has an easier time functioning and repairing itself, when needed.

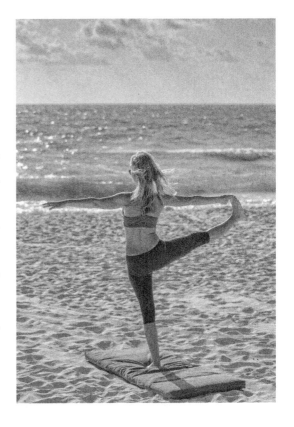

Yoga is extremely beneficial for aging bodies. It is a wonderful stress reliever as the motion is slow and fluid. Some poses are weight bearing, using your own weight, and so gently improve muscle quality while strengthening your bones. The poses help open up your entire body, allowing increased circulation, blood flow, and flexibility, which is imperative to maintain if you want to remain mobile and independent.

Performing yoga consistently will result in toned muscles from head to toe, reduce pain, improve flexibility and can reduce or eliminate back pain and nerve pain. Focusing on the right poses will also improve core strength, helping posture to remain intact with strong muscle balance. In addition, focusing on doing the moves and poses correctly is a form of mindfulness, which can result in an improved mind body connection, as well as stress relief.

Stretching can be used as an exercise routine, alone or with strength training. Stretching not only lengthens muscles, but causes you to use more surrounding muscle fibers of the main muscle you are working on, resulting in more power and strength. Just like in yoga, static stretching calls for the holding of poses to increase flexibility and agility. Most movements improve range of motion and circulation, and some find stretching routines to be easier than yoga poses.

Dynamic stretching utilizes motions that put joints and muscles through a whole range of motion, but without holding a stretch for any length of time. Exercises like the lunge or torso twist are forms of dynamic stretching, and should be done with care to avoid injuries. Whether you do dynamic or static stretching, most people find that practice makes the routine more enjoyable. After a couple of weeks, a stretching routine should feel more like a stress-break and less like exercise.

Thai Chi is another type of movement meditation that results in increased circulation, increased flexibility, improved balance and even lowered blood pressure. Some call Thai Chi the best exercise for balance and flexibility, and may be so since the slow, fluid movements are performed while standing.

The benefits of Thai Chi are posted in Biological Psychiatry, where the movements were found to reduce chronic inflammation. Another study showed that long-term use of Thai Chi slowed the decline of muscle strength in elderly people.[9] It also helps improve mood, as it can be used as a mindful meditation, as well.

✓ The Solution

Each of these exercises can be done at home or in a class. Yoga and Thai Chi classes are a great excuse to get out and meet others, but classes can be found online and for beginners, as well. Stretching classes have also become popular, or you can put together your own program.

---

9   Zhou M, Peng N, Dai Q, Li HW, Shi RG, Huang W. Effect of Tai Chi on muscle strength of the lower extremities in the elderly. Chin J Integr Med. 2016 Nov;22(11):861-866. doi: 10.1007/s11655-015-2104-7. Epub 2015 May 27. PMID: 26015074.

No matter which one you choose, be sure to incorporate movements that will use your entire body from head to toe. Go slowly because even though they seem static, overstretching or pulling the wrong way can result in tearing or pulling a muscle or ligament.

Foam Rolling

Foam rolling is used by many people to "roll" out the tension of a workout. But it can also be used to break up muscle fascia, allowing improved circulation and flexibility. And while most trainers teach to use a foam roller to reduce muscles soreness after a workout, there may be more to the benefits that that.

As we get older, our muscles and fascia become less pliable and resilient. Fascia is a type of covering or casing that surrounds muscles, and can actually bind to itself and lose elasticity. Myofascial release is a practice that is known to help separate the fibers and restore health and elasticity.

Foam rolling is a form of myofascial release. Releasing fascia is imperative to improve blood flow, collagen production, and oxygen to the muscles. Bound fascia traps and suffocates muscles and may even inhibit lymphatic flow. Many people feel discomfort and pain, at first, and the more pain you feel, the more "bound" your fascia.

At the same time, muscles could be hardened bands of tissue, due to inactivity, and the pain may not stem from the fascia, but instead from the bound of muscles bands.

A regular yoga practice can slow or even reverse the harmful effects of aging. Two new studies suggest that doing yoga regularly can slow physical aging and the harmful impact of stress at the cellular and DNA level.

169

The health of our fascia determines the state of our body as we age. Immobility is death for fascia. Lack of movement and increased pressure will stiffen it; when this happens, the fascia tends to glue together through a process called hydrogen bonding.

If your muscles are tight and "bound," exercise may induce cramping or pain that lasts for days. Foam rolling can help release muscles, bringing blood, nutrients and oxygen to them.

Foam rolling can help release connective tissue that becomes less pliable and elastic with age. Remember that as we get older, collagen and elastin are produced more slowly. The lack of elasticity can make it more difficult to move and choke off needed proteins that the body needs to help repair the tissue and replenish collagen. Not paying attention to all the connective tissue and muscles sets us up to fall into a cycle of accelerated aging.

✓ The Solution

A foam roller can be purchased online along with a guide on how-to do a routine. Many exercises can be found online for each area of the body. The concept is simple; with the foam roller on the floor, sit or place the area of your back, leg, or arm on the roller and slowly roll back and forth.

Foam rollers can be found in different sizes. If you are a beginner or not used to exercising, you might begin with a smaller diameter, so you can more easily support yourself without putting your full weight on the roller. Some rollers come with spongy protrusions to act more like a massage. Fortunately, they are not pricey, only around $20 for a roller, so purchasing a few different types can help you form an entire workout. You can also look into devices that are sold for Fascia Blasting. They are more expensive, but some people have gotten amazing results.

Lymphatic Drainage

Your body has a secondary circulatory system that is not made of blood, but of lymph. Lymph is a colorless fluid that contains white blood cells and toxins. Through lymph vessels, the fluid circulates through the body to pick up waste for neutralization or removal. It is an important part of your immune system and provides protection from pathogens to ward off disease. This is an extremely simple explanation for a complicated process, but for our needs this knowledge will suffice.

> "
> I love living. I love that I'm alive to love my age. There are many people who went to bed just as I did yesterday evening and didn't wake this morning. I love and feel very blessed that I did.
>
> **—Maya Angelou**

Unlike the cardiovascular system powered by the heart, the lymph does not have a pump. Instead, it relies on muscle contractions and manual movement for waste removal. Just like any system of your body, lymph circulation is also susceptible to slowing down, especially as we get older and less active.

When the lymphatic system doesn't move well, the fluid becomes stagnant. Just like any fluid that doesn't move, stagnancy can lead to thickness or crystallization and calcification, mainly in the lymph nodes, as they are not properly "cleansed" with healthy lymph fluid motion. This can cause problems such as a rise in lymph node disease and other serious conditions.

When lymph doesn't circulate efficiently, it becomes more difficult to filter pathogens and waste through the lymph nodes. White blood cells are not circulated as well, either, leaving you more susceptible to infection, impaired immune response, and diseases that can lead to accelerated aging. Paying attention to your lymphatic system can help you stay healthy and feel younger.

Lymphatic drainage is a way to deliberately help your body move lymph along. Since it relies on muscular contractions, massage helps as do the following practices.

✓ The Solution

- **Walking** is one of the best practices to move lymph. During a brisk walk, you contract muscles in your legs, torso or core, and arms. These miniscule contractions, along with increased blood circulation and oxygen intake help move the lymph, as well. Since you are exercising, you are performing two anti-aging hacks with one walk!

- **Mini Trampolines** are a fun way to exercise and assist with lymph drainage. As you bounce, your entire body is working against gravity, which helps build muscle. Jumping improves circulation, improves oxygen intake and causes muscular contractions throughout your entire body, thus forcing movement of the lymphatic fluid.

- **Pressotherapy** is a massage using a special suit, which inflates with air to apply pressure throughout the body. The computerized action stimulates the lymph much like manual lymphatic drainage does. This massage can be done in a spa or health center, or a suit and unit can be purchased for home use. The home devices are not very expensive. In fact, they probably cost the same as a series of treatments at the salon. If you have the space for this "space suit" and the will to use it regularly, you will experience amazing benefits, including a great improvement in cellulite and overall skin tone.

- **Dry Brushing,** used once or twice a week is a simple and affordable way to boost your lymphatic system and increase drainage. Simply buy a natural-bristle brush and just before your shower, starting from the knees brush upwards (always towards the heart), applying enough pressure to stimulate circulation.

With regular dry brushing you'll also increase blood circulation, promoting internal detoxification which can aid in weight loss, cellulite reduction and the elimination of accumulated toxins.

Get a Dog

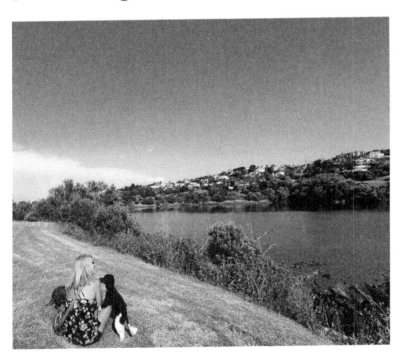

When it comes to home therapies, I saved the best for last… at least for animal lovers. Caring for a pet is a great way to motivate yourself to walk and enjoy life. Caring for a pet, like a dog, inspires many to get outside, go to a park, walk, run with the dog and play games. In fact, dog owners are four times as likely to meet physical activity guidelines than those who don't own a dog.

Dogs are a source of stress relief, non-judgmental, and offer unconditional love and emotional support. In fact, many dogs are specially trained to be support animals, as they can offer support and learn to do a multitude of tasks to take care of a human. Today, dogs help veterans, and many others cope with PTSD and improve stress management skills.

One study found that dogs are beneficial for heart health. In a review of studies over the span of 70 years, researchers concluded that dog owners had lower blood pressure and better stress response than those who are not dog owners.[10]

Pet therapy is being used in hospitals and nursing homes around the world. Interaction with dogs lessens agitated behavior in patients with dementia and improves cognitive function in patients with mental illness. It also lowers stress response in hospitalized patients who require long-term care. Imagine what a dog can do for your mind at home!

✓ The Solution

Research support dogs if you feel you have a special need or require special help at home. If not, go to your local shelter and rescue a dog. Rescue dogs are very grateful that you have saved their life, and will reward you with much love. Of course, only adopt if you have enough time to spend with your dog. As they're pack animals, being left home alone all day, every day, is absolute torture. A good alternative is to volunteer at a shelter to walk and cuddle the doggies when you have time.

---

10   Kramer, C., Caroline K. Kramer Caroline K. Kramer, Mehmood, S., Sadia Mehmood Leadership Sinai Centre for Diabetes (C.K.K., Suen, R., Renée S. Suen Leadership Sinai Centre for Diabetes (C.K.K., . . . Kazi, D. (2019, October 08). Dog Ownership and Survival. Retrieved November 05, 2020, from **https://www.ahajournals.org/doi/10.1161/ CIRCOUTCOMES.119.005554**

66

Aging happy and well, instead of sad and sick, is at least under some personal control. We have considerable control over our weight, our exercise, our education, and our abuse of cigarettes and alcohol. With hard work and therapy, our relationships with our spouses and our coping styles can be changed for the better. A successful old age may lie not so much in our stars and genes as in ourselves.

—George E. Vaillant

CHAPTER 6

Personal Practices

These are not truly "practices" as in setting aside time for exercise or following a particular diet. The hacks in this section are more like goals, and you must find the best way to try to reach the ones that resonate with you. But here, you will learn the importance of why some of these goals should be incorporated, or in some cases, left out. They can be surprisingly beneficial and help you in ways you never realized you needed.

Throw Away Your Spanx

I'm sure many women will not want to hear this, but please, throw away your Spanx or other type of constrictive shapewear. Restrictive clothing will interfere with digestive function and circulation of blood flow to certain organs. This can lead to a host of health issues that people may not relate to wearing restrictive clothing.

Restrictive wear has been around for centuries, including the rib breaking trend of corsets and gangrene inducing practice of foot binding for tiny feet. According to those in the medical community, restrictive shapewear is no different and can be harmful to your health. Check out some of the health issues they can cause:

- Irritated, red, itchy skin

- Tingling and numbness in legs due to compressed nerves

- Blood clots due to constricted circulation

- Poor digestion due to trapped gas, undigested food and compression of digestive organs

- Acid reflux due to constricted digestive tract

- Erosive Esophagitis due to compression that leads to disfunction of the valve that is supposed to prevent digestive juices from backing up the esophagus

Donning the too-tight shapewear every day can actually cause nerve damage, chronic pain, gastrointestinal problems and painful skin irritation.

- Yeast and bacterial infections

- Increase of pelvic organ prolapse (you will pee yourself more easily)

✓ The Solution

If you feel the need to use shapewear, perhaps a body detox or fast is in order. You will not only look better, but feel better and improve your overall health.

Keep in mind that intermittent fasting, detoxing with herbal supplements (such as for a liver cleanse) or water fasting will remove the excess weight and bloating around your midsection and hips. Also, it's important to note that every gram of carbs you eat (think bread, pasta, rice, etc.) will hold on to 3 grams of water. So the more carbs you're eating, the more water your body will retain, making you look and feel puffy and uncomfortable. The following are a few different ways to cleanse your body.

- Intermittent fasting will do wonders to reduce your waist size and promote the youthful growth hormone, the production of which significantly declines with age.

- Try an elimination diet to find out what foods may trigger bloating and gas in your body. Many vegetables, wheat, eggs and even dairy are often to blame.

- Do a 30-day Carnivore Diet for a total reset. This entails only eating meat and animal fat for 30 days. I've seen some amazing results when it comes to healing and weight loss just within these 30 days. After this, you can introduce eggs one week and then dairy the next week to see how your body reacts. You can then reintroduce vegetables one at a time if you like. You will quickly see which foods were causing the most issues. This is the ultimate elimination diet.

- Incorporate regular Water Fasts into your routine. Water Fasting can be as short as 24 hours or you can try longer fasts once you have more experience. This is a great way to cleanse your body, reset your metabolism and develop new healthier eating habits.

Please see my Water Fasting video for more info:

Channel: The Aging Games
How to Lose Weight with Water Fasting in 10 Days?

See my video for more info about Intermittent Fasting:

Channel: The Aging Games
Intermittent Fasting | 5 Common Mistakes that Prevent Weight Loss

Stimulate Your Vagus Nerve

The vagus nerve is the longest nerve in your body that is part of your autonomic nervous system, which is in charge of regulating metabolism, digestion, heart rate and other body functions that are unconsciously controlled. It is attached to your brain and travels through the neck onto your digestive system. It affects the heart, lungs, liver, spleen and pancreas. The activity of this nerve is often referred to as vagal tone and is the baseline measurement of activity.

While this might not mean much to us, you can think of it this way; high vagal tone is an indication that your body can relax quicker after a bout of stress. It is an indication of how you handle stress, overall. Having a high vagal tone reduces your risk of heart disease and stroke. You can enjoy lower blood pressure and improved digestion thanks to an increase in digestive enzymes.

I don't believe in aging. I believe in forever altering one's aspect to the sun.

—Virginia Woolf

But this nerve, often considered the source of "cross-talk" between your body systems and functions, can lose tone. Researchers and scientists point out that dysfunction of this nerve is due to hypoxia, or a disturbance in circulation, but there is more to it than this. Other research has found that many factors are responsible for the health of this nerve, from the gut microbiome to stress reduction practices like meditation.

Improving vagal tone helps create a positive cycle of health. High vagal tone increases positive emotions, which improves mental health leading to improved physical health (as happier people tend to take better care of themselves) which leads to an improved vagal tone, and the cycle continues. So, how can you stimulate your vagal nerve and enjoy improved tonality?

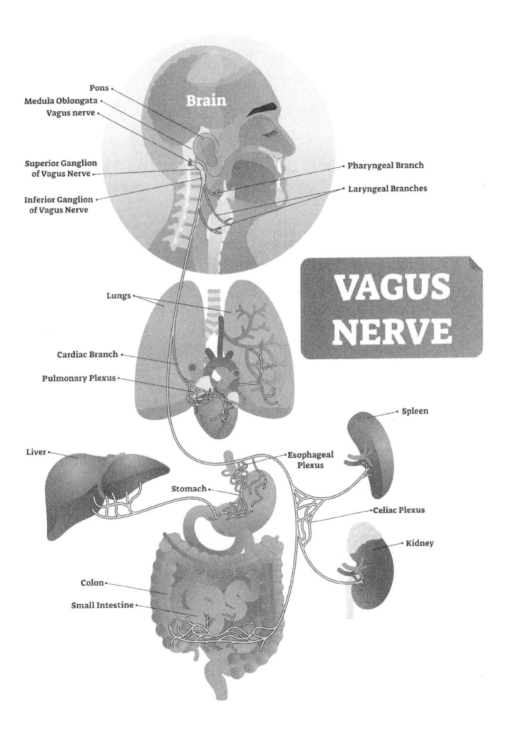

Pons
Medula Oblongata
Vagus nerve

Brain

Superior Ganglion
of Vagus Nerve

Pharyngeal Branch

Laryngeal Branches

Inferior Ganglion
of Vagus Nerve

Lungs

VAGUS NERVE

Cardiac Branch

Pulmonary Plexus

Spleen

Liver

Esophageal
Plexus

Stomach

Celiac Plexus

Kidney

Colon

Small Intestine

✓ The Solution

- Cold therapy increases parasympathetic activity through the vagal nerve, which improves vagal tone.

- Breathing therapy increases parasympathetic activity and reduces anxiety. Focus on long, slow breathing with longer exhales than inhales while relaxing your body with each exhale. For example, breathe in for 3 counts and out for 4, or any numbers that make you comfortable.

- Balance your gut microbiome to improve the function of the vagus nerve, which leads to improved brain function, as well. This can be done with probiotics, a healthy diet and cutting out sugar and other junk foods.

- Singing and humming creates vibrations that run the length of the vagus nerve, which can directly stimulate activity as you destress.

- Laugh as often as you can, because it stimulates your immune system along with the vagus nerve.

Improve Your Circadian Rhythm

The circadian rhythm is the cycle that our various bodily processes follow. Your sleep and digestive cycle both follow a set pattern over 24 hours. Hormonal cycles follow monthly patterns, for both men and women (and men go through their own monthly ups and downs and even have a form of "menopause"). Our hair grows in cycles and our skin sheds in cycles. It is important to keep our cycles in rhythm so our body functions at its best.

When the circadian rhythm is thrown out of sync, health problems can quickly follow. Studies show that eating late at night can lead to heart problems, obesity and metabolic issues.[1] Birth control is meant to help regulate women's menstrual cycles, while it does the exact opposite by disrupting the natural rhythm and eventually leading to health issues. People doing shift work increase their risk of cardiovascular disease by 40% according to studies. All three examples illustrate the importance of not messing up our natural cycles, but what more can we do?

First, it is helpful to understand that our circadian rhythm takes cues from our environment. For example, blue light can inhibit the stimulation of melatonin, a hormone necessary to induce sleep. Other hormones also play roles such as cortisol from stress can interrupt sleep as can alcohol and diet. Medications, poor sleep habits, travel and stress can all interfere with our natural circadian rhythm. But the good news is that you can fix it.

✓ The Solution

Lifestyle changes can help improve your circadian rhythm and get you back on track with a healthy cycle that supports health.

- Try a few seconds of sungazing every morning when the sun rises. This sun exposure on your retina will signal the pineal gland to make melatonin at night. Melatonin is an important hormone made during dark hours that helps us sleep.

- In combination with sun gazing, you can also take a brisk walk outside shortly after you get up in the morning. The sunshine will signal your hormones that it's time to wake up and make some vitamin D.

- Contrary to what you've heard your whole life, breakfast is NOT the most important meal of the day. Any time you can comfortably skip

---

1   Kinsey AW, Ormsbee MJ. The health impact of nighttime eating: old and new perspectives. Nutrients. 2015;7(4):2648-2662. Published 2015 Apr 9. doi:10.3390/nu7042648

Aging reduces the ability to benefit from sun stimulation through the eyes, mostly due to eye-related diseases such as glaucoma and cataracts. Chronic inflammation and carbohydrate intolerance are two common problems associated with these, as well as other eye disorders.

breakfast, you are increasing the window within which your body is fasting.

- Exercise during the day to increase oxygen and circulation and to reduce stress. Regular, daily exercise will also help you sleep better at night. Check out the book *In the Flo* by Alisa Vitti for the best types of exercises to do during different stages of your cycle. For example, more gentle exercises are best during menstruation, such as walking, while HIIT is most effective mid cycle. You can expect to lose more weight and gain muscle more easily when you sync your exercise routine with your cycle.

- Eat your largest meal of the day mid-day, when your digestion and digestive enzymes are at their peak.

- Keep your home bright with natural sunlight throughout the day, or try to be near natural sunlight at work.

- Eat a light dinner in the evening so you don't tax your digestive system. Avoid eating after sunset if you can.

- Have a bedtime routine that includes relaxing practices like taking a lavender bath, meditation or reading. Try to avoid blue light for at least a couple of hours before bed. Use blue blockers and candles at night.

- Sleep in complete darkness so you don't disturb your sleep hormone cycle.

- Try a melatonin supplement when traveling across different time zones.

Rewire Your Brain

Rewiring your brain is based in the brain's ability to constantly form new pathways for electrical and thought signals to travel through. The process is called plasticity and is a function that helps us learn and adjust to new environments.

The problem with brain connections takes place during negative incidents. One traumatic or perceived traumatic event can cause a series of connections that your brain relies on to predict future outcomes. For example, if a teacher with brown hair wearing a brown dress embarrasses you in front of classmates for eating an orange in class, you might find yourself feeling anxious each time you meet a woman with brown hair wearing a brown dress, or you might find you hate oranges. This basic description hardly covers how in-depth the process is, but you get the idea.

> With age comes the inner, the higher life. Who would be forever young, to dwell always in externals?
>
> **—Elizabeth Cady Stanton**

Our brains form connections through our entire lives, and the more they use the same connections, the more reinforced a pathway will become. As one famous twentieth century psychologist said, "Neurons that fire together, wire together." This is how habits are formed and why they are sometimes difficult to break. This can also stop us from seeing the truth about a person or situation, as we color them with glasses from past incidents and only hear or see what we expect to hear and see.

The good thing is that you can use neuroplasticity to change your connections and see the world in a whole different light. Learning a new

The great thing about getting older is that you become more mellow. Things aren't as black and white, and you become much more tolerant. You can see the good in things much more easily rather than getting enraged as you used to do when you were young.

—**Maeve Binchy**

game, traveling to new places, meeting new people and trying new foods will all stimulate your brain to build new connections. Just to give you an example, as you're driving home from work on the same route you've done a million times, your brain is pretty much on autopilot. You don't really have to think too much about it. Now compare this to being in a new city and driving around trying to find a place you've never been to before. This is when your brain is in overdrive trying to process all the new info and visuals. The good news is that it's never too late to form new neurons, and there are some very deliberate ways to help rewire your brain in a positive way.

✓The Solution

Music is one way to help rewire your brain. This method is so powerful that music therapy is used today to slow cognitive decline in older people, can improve mood, coordination, and even strengthen memory.

Some music includes subliminal messages or binaural beats to enhance brain function. Others include instruments that are traditionally used for meditation like the spirit drum, singing bowls and Koshi chimes. You can even listen to these while sleeping.

Frequencies measure brainwaves, and different brainwaves are associated with different levels of consciousness. Alpha waves are associated with awake but restful states during activities like praying or reading, beta waves are associated with daily waking hours where you are doing tasks that require your attention, theta waves occur during deep relaxation or sleeping and delta waves occur during deep sleep or deep meditation. Using practices like meditation and neurofeedback can help you train your brain to use the different frequencies to your advantage.

Exercise that is varied and takes place in different locations can oxygenate the brain and promote brain growth factors. Try not to get caught up in the same routine day after day. The body, and especially the brain, loves variety.

Challenge your mind by tackling puzzles, games, and stimulating but fun intellectual tasks.

Use Natural Cosmetics

Regular cosmetics can be highly toxic and lead to skin conditions like redness or itching while accelerating the aging process of your skin, instead of making you look younger. Many of these products contain harmful chemicals that can enter the bloodstream and wreak havoc on your health and hormones. Some may also include unregulated chemicals and highly questionable ingredients. This happens because there are tens of thousands of chemicals used in the environment today, most of which go unregulated.

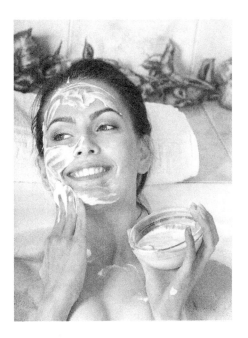

When it comes to cosmetics, some experts estimate the average person puts around 515 individual chemicals on their face each day, including washes, astringents, creams, serums, and cosmetics. Add to this perfumes, cleaners you come into contact with, body washes, lotions and more, and it becomes easy to see how this happens. Some toxic chemicals include:

- Formaldehyde - can cause irritation of the eyes, nose, and throat, even at low levels and have been linked to cancers such as leukemia.

- Mercury - may have toxic effects on the nervous, digestive and immune systems, and on lungs, kidneys, skin and eyes.

- Methylene glycol (a form of formaldehyde)—long-term exposure may lead to kidney failure and brain damage

- Quaternium 15 (releases formaldehyde)—common ingredient in shampoos and soaps, an allergen that can cause contact dermatitis in susceptible individuals.

- Isobutyl and isopropyl parabens (hormone disruptor) - parabens are believed to disrupt hormone function by mimicking estrogen. Too much estrogen can trigger an increase in breast cell division and growth of tumors, which is why paraben use has been linked to reproductive issues and breast cancer.

- M- and O-phynylenediamine in hair dyes (can damage DNA and cause cancer) - may cause severe dermatitis, eye irritation and tearing, asthma, gastritis, renal failure, vertigo, tremors, convulsions, and coma in humans. Eczematoid contact dermatitis may result from chronic exposure in humans.

- Phthalates (hormone disruptors) - can damage the liver, kidneys, lungs, and reproductive system. Also been linked to asthma, ADHD, breast cancer, obesity and type II diabetes, low IQ, behavioral issues and fertility issues.

- Sodium lauryl sulfate - a detergent used in cosmetics, is a skin, eye and respiratory tract irritant and toxic to aquatic organisms. It is a common ingredient in shampoos, but it can strip natural oils from the scalp and hair, thus making it more dry and brittle.

Because of the chemical world we live in, it becomes more important that we try to control what we do put on our skin.

It starts even before birth! Of the 287 chemicals detected in umbilical cord blood, we know that 180 cause cancer in humans, 217 are toxic to the brain and nervous system, and 208 cause birth defects or abnormal development in animal tests.

√The Solution

- The Environmental Working Group (EWG) has an online tool called The Healthy Living App, which is a guide to identify safer personal care products. When the app is installed on your phone, go to the Cosmetics tab and scan the bar code to see their safety rating.

- Read labels to avoid "red flag" ingredients like synthetic fragrance, parabens, triclosan, formaldehyde, oxybenzone, denatured alcohol, and anything petroleum derived.

- Seek out organic, natural, cosmetic and makeup brands with V (vegan), O (organic) and S (sustainable)

- Try to learn about the companies you purchase from. Smaller companies seem to have more integrity when it comes to using toxic versus non-toxic ingredients.

There are more than 7,000 chemicals in cigarette smoke. More than 70 of those chemicals are linked to cancer.

- Develop a skin care routine that incorporates natural ingredients to create a healthy and glowing complexion.

Stop Smoking

Smoking can be fatal, and if not, it can certainly interfere with your energy, health and appearance. Those who smoke often have a certain smell of stale smoke or nicotine, and also noticeably deeper lines and wrinkles, including the small wrinkles that form around the mouth from pursing the lips. Smoking also discolors the teeth, which can make one look older than her years.

As we mature and our immune system slows down, we must work harder to keep it stimulated. Unfortunately, smoking makes this more difficult as we inhale carcinogens that are known to cause numerous types of cancer including mouth, throat, lungs, stomach, liver and bowel.

Smoking damages the heart and can increase the sticky plaque buildup that leads to heart disease, stroke and damaged blood vessels. It raises blood pressure, reduces the supply of blood to the brain and damages lung tissue. It can cause impotence in men. This is a lot of reasons to stop smoking!

✓The Solution

If you are an avid smoker, try stopping at certain times of the day. For example, if you smoke first thing in the morning, try waiting 30 minutes before your first cigarette. After a week, wait 60 minutes, and so on. Take your time in steps and it will become a habit to not smoke.

Many people associate their first cigarette with a cup of coffee and find it difficult to stop. If this is you, then find other parts of the day to make it a habit to stop. Try not smoking during work, when socializing, or at dinner time. Slowly widen the gaps so you don't have much smoking time left. It will become a habit to not smoke, although it takes time.

Stop cold turkey if you can. This means just put them down and don't look back. Most people quit like this, especially during illness. It is highly effective, although may be uncomfortable at first. Replace cigarettes with healthy habits like walking, dancing, or reading. Do anything to distract your mind from smoking.

We don't grow older, we grow riper.

—**Pablo Picasso**

Neutral Makeup for a Younger Appearance

Did you know that makeup actually ages people? Even those who are young will look older when they slather makeup on their faces. A five-year-old girl can easily look like a short 20-year-old, and a 12-year-old girl can appear to be 30 years of age with the right makeup! Keep this in mind when applying your own makeup.

Makeup can bring out all the fine lines and wrinkles of every area of the face.

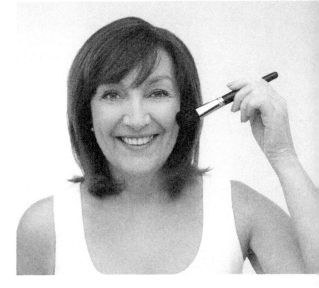

Black eyeliner will accentuate bags and wrinkles around the eyes while making them appear smaller. This is an issue because as we age, our eyes do get smaller. The only way to combat that is through the previously mentioned facial exercises, and by not accentuating it with black eyeliner.

Avoid bright red lipstick. As we age, our lips become smaller and wrinkles may form around them due to smoking and lots of laughing and talking. Again, some facial exercises can address this to an extent. So, what should mature people do for makeup? Keep it neutral for a fresh, youthful and natural look!

✓ The Solution

- Go barefaced as much as you can, allowing your skin to breathe freely

- Use only natural, organic makeup

- Get a lesson on how to best apply makeup for your age, skin type and features

- Use a primer so foundation goes on smoothly

- Wear a foundation close to your natural skin color; some beauty experts recommend going a shade warmer, so you don't appear "washed out"

- Use a concealer for dark circles only if you need to and be sure it doesn't accentuate lines or wrinkles

- Use a bronzer around your face to warm your skin tone and help it glow

- Smile and apply light, muted rose colored blush for a natural color

- Be careful when applying mascara as clumpy eyelashes can age you

- Don't go too dark on the eyebrows, aim for a natural, brushed look

- Use a lip liner pencil to give mature lips more definition, then apply matching lipstick or gloss in a neutral or muted shade, blend it with the liner for a natural look

Check out my video about eyebrow tattooing:

Channel: The Aging Games
Microblading Eyebrows Before and After
Experience

Brows are back! Not only are full brows totally trendy, but they can also help give an overall more youthful look. You can use eyebrow pencils or permanent make-up for a longer-term solution.

Ditch the Sunglasses

While the experts have told us for years that sunlight can kill you, it turns out lack of sunlight is far more harmful. It can lead to osteoporosis, cancer and depression. And it turns out that sunscreen can cause cancer instead of preventing it. So, what does that mean for our eyes?

Certain shades can increase the amount of harmful radiation the eyes are exposed to. This can lead to retinal tissue damage, cataracts and macular degeneration, all symptoms of aging. These are often the reasons that manufacturers of some sunglasses tell people to get them to pay more for their expensive sunglasses. But I believe we should ditch them altogether, and here's why:

- Firstly, the above is true. Wearing sunglasses without the proper protection can be worse than wearing none

Sungazing should be done for a few seconds only. Safe times are the first hour after sunrise, and the last hour before sunset. When you sungaze, it's best to be barefoot, standing on grass or the ground.

at all. This is because the glasses can prevent your pupils from dilating and allow even more harmful UV light in.

- Wearing sunglasses makes your eyes lazy with less ability to adapt to dark and light. Your eyes use muscles to open and close the pupil and even to elongate and shorten as you look far away or close up. And just like any other muscle, if you don't use it, you lose it. In this case, its loss of adaptive abilities.

- Our eyes are naturally made to work in sunlight. Wearing sunglasses causes your eyes to work in an unnatural way as it tries to adjust the colors. This can lead to eye fatigue and stress.

- You don't want to burn? Ditch the sunglasses! When wearing glasses your eyes send a signal to your brain that it's a cloudy day, thus not preparing your skin for strong UV rays and tanning.

- When sunlight enters our eyes, it stimulates the hypothalamus, and areas of the brain that are connected to the pineal gland and helps regulate the sleep cycle.

- There's no other creature on the planet that uses a fake apparatus to shield its eyes from the sun. We were made to live in perfect harmony with nature.

Improve Your Eyesight

Many people don't realize that we can not only improve but actually heal our vision. Most of us have been indoctrinated our entire lives that if you have poor eyesight, you need eyeglasses or contact lenses to help you see better. In reality, when you look far away, close up, or in between, your eyeballs change shape accordingly.

The above description is a theory by Dr. William Bates (1860 - 1930) and goes against the mainstream theory of the Helmholtz theory, which is still in use today. In his theory, tiny ciliary muscles in the lens of the eye change the thickness of the lens to allow one to focus.

These two theories are important to understand why eye exercises may or may not work. In the Bates theory, muscles are responsible for changing eye shape that helps us focus. In the Helmholtz theory, the thickness of the lens simply wears out or becomes unusable for some reason, and fixing it is beyond our abilities.

Dr. Bate's theory is a positive and empowering theory that puts faith in the adaptability and resilience of the human body. He postulates that the recovery of good vision is possible and that the eyes change all the time, in relation to our environment, lifestyle, emotional state and habits.

Thankfully, tens of thousands of people around the world have successfully used the Bates method to improve their eyesight. The method does not stop at

Doctors won't make you healthy. Nutritionists won't make you slim. Teachers won't make you smart. Gurus won't make you calm. Mentors won't make you rich. Trainers won't make you fit. Ultimately, you have to take responsibility. Save yourself.

—Naval Ravikant

To relieve eye strain, every 20 minutes, look away from your computer or phone screen for at least 20 seconds and direct your gaze to an object that's at least 20 feet away.

simply near or farsightedness, but includes healing from any other issues like stigmatism and presbyopia. More exciting, those that use the Bate's method have found a new clarity in vision they never had before; colors appear brighter, more awareness of their surroundings and more vivid dreams. The great thing is that we can all use the Bates method any time we like.

✓ The Solution

Luckily for all of us, Dr. Bates was very generous with his teaching and guides, for the Bate's method can be purchased or found for free online. Many people hold classes at local annexes to teach how to do them, and you can easily incorporate them into your daily life.

Today, with so many people having so much success with eye exercises, there are many hybrids and similar methods based on the Bate's method. Search around and give it a try to enjoy better vision and to use your eyes more, which will help them adapt and keep them young at any age.

Check out this video for more info:

Channel: Nathan Oxenfeld
Bates Method 101: What Is The Bates Method?

Smile

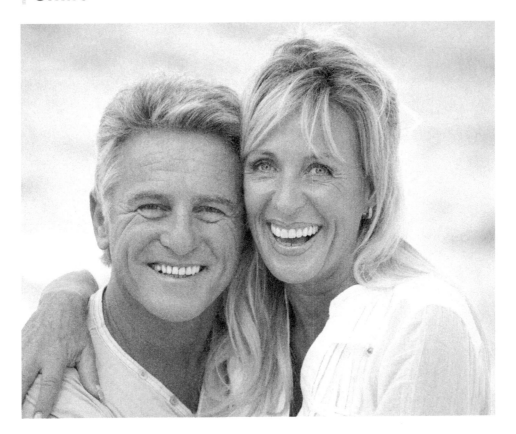

As we get older, it's no secret that gravity has an effect on our facial skin. But smiling can provide an instant facelift and brighten your outlook on life! It may sound superficial, but there are psychological reasons as well as aesthetic reasons to smile.

Each of our faces age differently, that is a given. But some things are common, including the downward droop of the corners of the mouth. Add to this the droopy eyebrows and eyelids and it is easy to fall into looking like an angry old person, no matter how happy you feel inside. When you look angry, people will naturally treat you differently. Here are more reasons to smile:

Researchers found that people who smile are often perceived as being younger than their actual age, while people who frown appear to be older than they really are.

- You will feel happier, almost instantly

- Smiling can lower your blood pressure as you feel more relaxed

- Smiling and laughing is a great stress reliever, and less stress can make anyone look younger

- Smiling can increase your body's ability to fight infection

- Smiling and laughing releases endorphins, which are natural pain relievers

✓ The Solution

Smile and laugh as often as you can!

Learn Gratitude

Learning to be grateful is a powerful way to improve health, both physically and mentally. To learn gratitude is to acknowledge the good in your life, the good in those around you and the good in the world. It is being thankful for your own health, skills, and talents. Recognizing the good around us even helps neuroplasticity, so your brain sees the good things, and will soon recognize even more, which will improve emotional and mental health.

Practicing gratitude can be as easy as remembering to say thank you, or to see the good in the people around you such as your partner or children. When you practice gratitude, you might find your relationships improve and work becomes more enjoyable. You will experience less stress, which will have a positive impact on your physical and mental health. And your happiness score will increase!

✓The Solution

Practicing gratitude can be done in many ways. Keeping a journal and adding to it each day can help it feel more tangible. Others prefer to pray each day and include a mental evaluation of everything they are grateful for. Still others begin the day by creating a mental list of everything to be grateful for before they get out of bed. And addressing different areas of your life that you are thankful for will impact your brain in different ways.

Taking a mental evaluation and listing things you are thankful for from your childhood or younger years can help you change a negative perspective of your history into a positive one. Listing all the things you are grateful for right now, in your present experience, can help you have a more positive outlook on life and see more opportunities as they come to you. And looking to the future with a positive spin while being grateful for the current gifts, talents or opportunities that can get you there can help you create a better future.

Meditate Daily

Meditation for inner health, vibrating youth and positivity is an incredibly effective tool for anti-aging. As a powerful stress reducer, daily meditation has been shown to help lower blood pressure, improve sleep and memory skills.

Studies have found that grateful people experience a number of health benefits - all associated with a more radiance, younger complexion.

It promotes a healthy outlook on life and has been used for centuries to slow the aging process of monks around the world.

Today, stress might be one of the quickest ways to accelerate aging. Studies have shown that chronic, ongoing stress affects our health and is linked to high blood pressure, diabetes, obesity, depression and heart disease. It interferes with hormones and deteriorates the gut microbiome. Physical stress shows on the face as increased frown lines, downturned mouth, and increased "marionette lines," that run from the side of the mouth toward the chin. One study even showed how the telomeres of mothers who cared for a chronically sick child were shorter than mothers whose children were not sick, showing how stress can shorten our lifespan.[2]

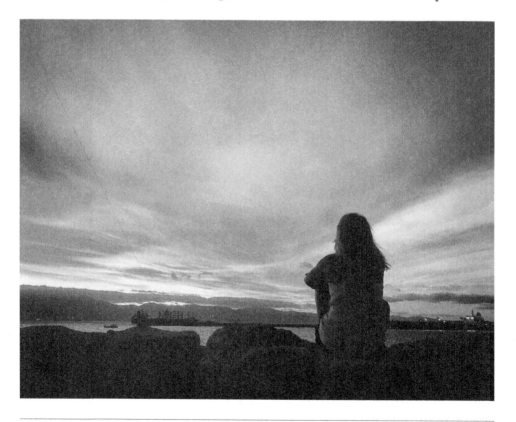

2   Aging, Chronic Disease and Telomeres Are Linked in Recent Studies. (2020, November 04). Retrieved November 06, 2020, from **https://www.ucsf.edu/news/2011/02/103672/aging-chronic-disease-and-telomeres-are-linked-recent-studies**

See my video on the 5 top reasons to meditate:

Channel: The Aging Games
5 Benefits of Meditation for Optimal Health and Wellbeing

Many people believe that being happier helps slow down the aging process. Meditation reduces feelings of anxiety and improves your overall emotional health.

Begin today to slow or reverse the aging process of your mind and body through regular meditation. Begin with just five minutes each day and work your way into more time when it is possible. Here are just some reasons why daily meditation is important:

- Meditation increases telomerase production, which helps rebuild telomeres after cells divide

- Those who meditate increase their lifespan by at least 10%

- Better sleep

- Lowered blood pressure

- Better stress response

- Less anxiety

- Less facial lines and wrinkles

- Healthy glow and complexion

Please check out my video to help slow down aging through meditation:

Channel: The Aging Games
Slow and Reverse Aging with this Guided Meditation and
Healing 528hz Music

✓ The Solution

Learning to meditate is easy, and practice increases the benefits fairly quickly. While there are a variety of methods for meditation, the following is a straightforward method.

Sit comfortably in a quiet and semi dark space, with your back straight. Some people believe you must sit with your legs crossed on the floor, but it is not necessary. Sitting on a chair, sofa or even the edge of your bed with both feet on the ground and your back straight (with a focus on a strong core) will suffice. The use of no back rest is to help you not fall asleep. If you prefer to meditate lying down, that's also fine.

1. Begin by doing your best to clear your mind and focus on your breathing.

2. Take notice of your body and ensure it is as relaxed as possible throughout the meditation. Of course some muscles will be supporting your frame to sit upright, but you can relax the muscles around those.

3. Count your breaths; either count to 3 on each inhale and then 4 on each exhale, or simply count your breaths in a series of 4 (1,2,3,4,1,2,3,4, etc.).

4. The goal is to only think of your breathing and nothing else. When something else enters your mind, gently clear it and regain focus on your breathing.

5. Set a timer for 5 or 10 minutes for the first week. Increase your time as it feels natural.

6. Feel free to set crystals around you, play meditation music, dab on essential oils, or include any other tool that will help you relax and focus.

7. You can also try a guided meditation to get you started.

Check out my video for beginner's learning to meditate:

Channel: The Aging Games
Learn to Meditate | Guided Meditation for Beginners

Buteyko Breathing for Health

Buteyko breathing is a breathing exercises created to help you take in less oxygen. This might sound counterintuitive, but there is a definite science behind it. When we are stressed, we breathe short and shallow, resulting in many breaths over the course of an hour or a day. Many people do this all day without realizing it. Doing so increases oxygen intake, but does not include enough balance of an exhale or pause to allow a sufficient amount of carbon dioxide to process the oxygen. This results in less ability to utilize the oxygen that we do inhale. Quite often, people make up for the lack of oxygen by breathing through the mouth, which can negatively affect the quality of our breathing and sleep patterns.

Learning to breathe properly allows more oxygen to be taken into the bloodstream and used throughout the body. Many people using the Buteyko Method report that it helps with asthma, anxiety, and sleep disorders. As we get older, it becomes more difficult to sleep through the night, and anxiety increases. Practicing this method can help you breathe in more oxygen with less exertion and improve your sleep and overall health.

Check out my video about Buteyko for more info:

Channel: The Aging Games
Buteyko Breathing Exercises - Everything you Need to Know about the Buteyko Method

✓The Solution

There are 7 exercises to this breathing method, here I will briefly cover one. The goal is to breathe through your nostrils only during the day and during sleep.

1. Relax and place your finger under your nose, horizontally. It should partially block the passageway, allowing air to enter only through the nostril tips.

2. Reduce the volume of air you breathe in by only breathing in lightly

3. When you exhale, count the seconds. Relax in this pause of the exhale as long as you can, comfortably.

4. Do your best to remain relaxed during the process.

5. Do this for 3-5 minutes, then take a 5-minute break and repeat 3 more times.

Here's a video of another exercise you can do with my friend Britta:

Channel: The Aging Games
Buteyko Breathing Exercises to Learn How to Breathe the Buteyko Way

Essential Oils (Aromatherapy)

Essential oils are a luxurious way to experiment with an alternative method of healing, balancing and mindfulness. They are extremely versatile and have been used by traditional healers for centuries, with records of use dating back to biblical times and Ancient Egypt. Oils are available for uses from healing, stress relief, lung health to beauty care, hormonal balance and more. Additionally, essential oils are a beautiful addition to a bath or meditation.

Essential oils are plant oils derived from the flowers, stems or leaves of plants, and the part used depends on which type of oil it is. Once distilled, the oils take on the scent of the plant oils and retain powerful healing properties. Some of the more popular oils and uses include:

- Lavender for stress relief

- Bergamot for eczema

- Jasmine for improved mood and to fight depression

Breathing through the nose peacefully balances levels of nitric oxide, carbon dioxide and oxygen in the body, calms the nervous system, boosts immunity, clears the mind, improves focus and increases overall energy.

205

- Rose for youthful skin and to balance Testosterone (important for both sexes) and is also known as an aphrodisiac and can aid libido

- Tea tree oil to kill fungus

- Chamomile for stress reduction

- Ginger for nausea

- Clary Sage for relaxation and to relieve hot flashes during menopause

- Sweet orange to reduce stress

- Peppermint for alertness, nausea and headaches

- Frankincense to balance thyroid hormones (T3 and T4) and to lower cortisol

- Thyme can have a positive effect on female hormones by increasing progesterone

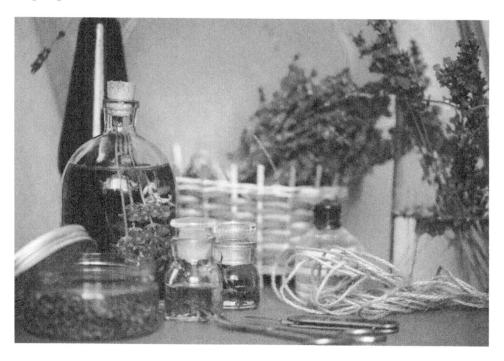

Some oils like lemon, lavender, peppermint, orange and tea tree oil have been shown to help kill bacteria, fungus and other harmful microbes. Lemon oil is more effective at killing bacteria than chemical spray cleaners, and prevents bacterial strains from mutating, unlike chemical disinfectants. Many people today are moving away from using so many chemicals in their homes and take advantage of these microbial properties for a number of uses.

✓ The Solution

When you use essential oils on your skin, always dilute it with a carrier oil or it can discolor or irritate your skin. Carrier oils include almond, olive, coconut, jojoba, argan or grapeseed oil. The following is a list of ways to use essential oils. Remember, they are also very powerful when used in combination.

- Add lavender to your laundry with your soap to freshen it

- Use lemon, grapefruit or orange oil with vinegar for a homemade cleaning solution

- Add a few drops of the oil of your choice in your bath

- Add a drop of rose oil to your daily face cream

- Citronella oil can be used to ward off mosquitos and bugs, especially when combined with vanillin

- Add a few drops of oil to an aromatherapy diffuser so the whole family can enjoy the benefits

- Add a drop or two of lavender oil mixed with a carrier oil onto an injury before covering to promote healing

One study found that frankincense was effective in reducing the appearance of scarring and stretch marks on a person's skin. It may have the same effect on wrinkles and fine lines.

- Apply a couple of drops of peppermint oil to the temples to relieve a migraine

- Use tea tree oil directly on your toenails to treat stubborn fungus

Use aromatherapy during meditation by applying a diluted oil to your skin or use in an aromatherapy diffuser.

Play Brain Games

Mental decline happens to everyone as we age. But you can slow the process by playing games that stimulate your brain and keep you young, engaged and active. Games are a form of brain training that can improve cognitive functions including better memory, response time, problem solving and logic. There are games that work different areas of the brain in order to stimulate its ability to rewire itself as needed.

Recall that neuroplasticity is a process of rewiring that the brain is always doing. As with any body function, the process slows down as we age. But we can stimulate the process with games, which promote new connections and pathways. These new pathways encourage more blood and oxygen into the brain and we now have a cycle of a healthy brain instead of a declining one.

✓ The Solution

The best way to stimulate your brain is to keep it active with a variety of activities, such as

- Learn or play chess or checkers

- Play Sudoku

- Learn card games and play them regularly

- Read both fiction and non-fiction books

- Put together puzzles

- Write in a journal and try your hand at creative writing

- Do crossword puzzles

- Get a math workbook and do the exercises

- Find online resources for games with the ability to track your progress, including: Brangle, Luminosity, Happy Neuron and Elevate

Brain stimulating memory games and puzzles for adults have long been known to have huge health benefits. They help keep one's mind active, the memory sharp, and they can slow down and even reverse the aging process.

Go Camping

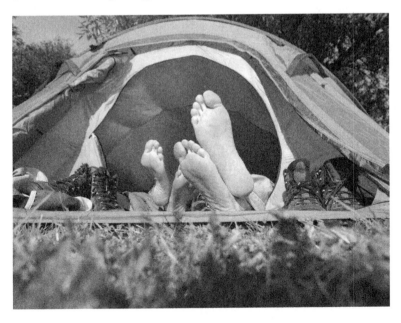

Camping has a number of health benefits from improving your mood, clearing your lungs by filling them with fresh air, reducing stress levels, increasing exercise, exposure to sunshine and even socialization. One of the most overlooked benefits of camping it that it can help you reset your biological clock.

Our circadian rhythms depend on nature for cues to produce certain hormones, such as melatonin for sleep. We require sunlight for a variety of health reasons; from making vitamin D to improved mental health. Living indoors may be harming us in more ways than we think, but we can undo some damage and mitigate further damage by camping on a regular basis.

One fascinating report was published in Current Biology, in which a group of volunteers were monitored while camping. Camping took place for one week during winter, with the least sunlight per day. Campers were only allowed natural daylight and light from a campfire at night. Light levels were recorded with special watches and blood tests monitored melatonin, the sleep hormone.

The most incredible finding was that the volunteers were exposed to 13 times more natural light during this winter camping escapade than when home. Campers were able to produce more melatonin earlier and go to bed sooner. Waking time was in tune with a healthy 24-hour cycle. Keep in mind campers had no access to phones or television, either, so it was concluded that filling the day with more natural sunlight with less unnatural light exposure at night can help us remain in a healthy circadian rhythm and cycle.

✓ The Solution

- Try camping once a month or every weekend, if possible

- If you cannot camp, choose a weekend to spend the days outdoors, avoid phone and television use and use candlelight or moonlight at night

- Take off your shoes and spend some time grounded to the Earth while camping

- Sit around a fire and talk about ghost stories

- You can have a virtual camping session in your backyard as well

- Have fun with it in the process!

Correct Your Posture

Posture can say a lot about how we feel. A hunched over posture can signal fatigue, illness or defeat. A tall, rigid posture can indicate we are overly rigid or frightened. A tall and relaxed posture can indicate confidence. No matter what your posture says about you, poor posture can lead to pain and disease. Learning to correct it will have both mental and physical benefits.

Good posture can keep your spine youthful, so you feel and look younger. Your blood, lymph, and spinal fluid can all flow more effortlessly, allowing more oxygen and nutrients to travel throughout your body. You will experience less back pain and your muscles will strengthen to

> *The anti-aging benefits of being connected to nature cannot be overlooked. Camping is a great way to destress, rejuvenate and charge your batteries, all of which will improve your overall wellbeing and appearance.*

help support your newfound stance. Here are some other benefits of correcting your posture:

- Less headaches

- More energy

- Less premature wearing of joints

- Increased lung capacity

- Improved digestion

- Improved circulation

When sitting, your feet should be flat on the floor. Keep your spine straight but relaxed and ensure your weight is distributed evenly on both hips.

Standing posture is tall and straight, while relaxed. Standing with your back against a wall with your head touching the wall can give you an idea of how "off" your posture is. Correct posture will not be your entire spine and head touching the wall, but instead your lower back, knees and head will not touch.

✓ The Solution

- Avoid walking with your head leading the way, as this can eventually lead to a sore neck and spine.

- Use a foam roller to roll out your mid back

- Strengthen your core with exercise

- Gently stretch your neck every day

- Improve your posture by imagining a silver cord that goes through your spine and out the top of your head. In your imagination, gently pull the silver cord from the top to straighten you up.

- Pay attention to your body when you stand and walk, to learn where any postural weakness exists, is so you can strengthen it

- Hold books and devices at eye level so you're not forced to look down on them (this will stop early jowls from forming as well)

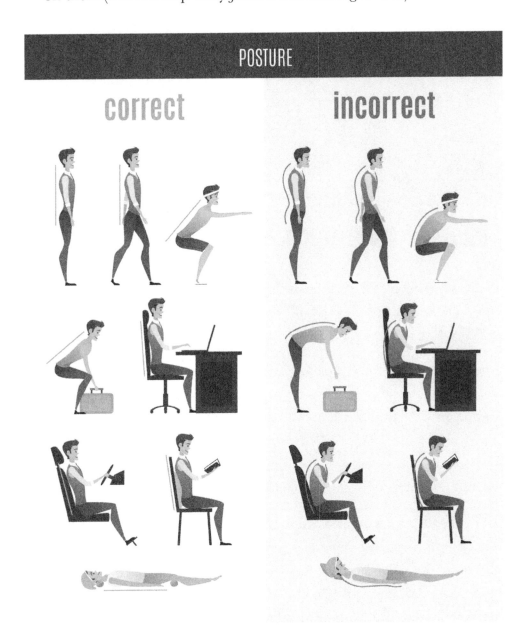

Get Your Boobies in the Sun

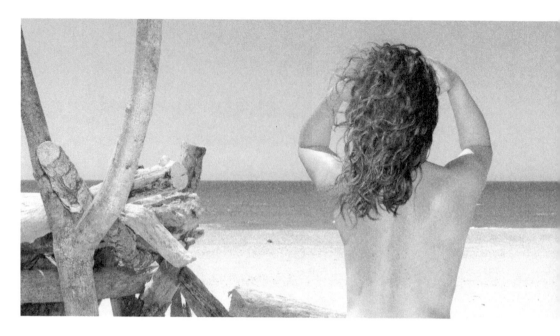

Neurosurgeon Jack Kruse has studied breast cancer extensively to find the mechanism that lies behind why so many women succumb to the disease. And what he found was very interesting, and backed by research.

Our breasts need to be exposed to sunlight on a regular basis, and those with the least exposure have an exponentially higher chance of breast tumor growth. Earlier I mentioned that we need sunlight so our bodies can manufacture vitamin D, but sunlight also helps the body manufacture natural progesterone, a hormone required in the delicate balance of hormones we need to remain healthy and cancer-free.

If we don't get enough vitamin D, we will also experience altered estradiol (an estrogen hormone), and altered testosterone. Sun also helps the body optimize vitamin A, which helps convert certain cholesterols into pregnenolone, another hormone required in the vast network of natural hormones that are crucial for our bodily functions. At this point you should be able to see how it becomes nearly impossible to medically balance hormones, and this is only a tip of the iceberg.

Dr. Kruse found in his research that a photopigment called melanopsin is bound to vitamin A and lack of sun creates melanopsin dysfunction, further degrading our hormonal balance. He also reported that exposure of mammary glands to sunlight literally inhibited oncogenesis (tumor development), ensuring estrogen and testosterone levels remain healthy.

The bottom line is that Dr. Kruse has taught for years that breast cancer is a result of an unhealthy circadian rhythm caused by lack of sunlight. Today, there is research from a study at Texas AM that links breast cancer to circadian rhythm.[3] Perhaps this quote by Dr. Kruse is true, "The sun is nature's vaccine for breast cancer."

✓ The Solution

Expose your breasts to the sun (without sunscreen) to ensure the necessary vitamins are synthesized and the hormonal processes fall into place that are required to prevent breast cancer. Luckily, partial exposure of your breasts should suffice if you are not in a place to go full nude. There are also tan-through bathing suits that you can wear so you can expose your breasts to the sun discretely in public. Keep in mind that vitamin D supplements may not mimic all the benefits the sun has to offer.

---

3   Scienmag. (2018, May 8). Texas A&M study links breast cancer to the body's internal clock: Scienmag: Latest Science and Health News. Retrieved November 07, 2020, from **https://scienmag.com/texas-am-study-links-breast-cancer-to-the-bodys-internal-clock/**

CHAPTER 7

Spa & Medical Treatments

The following treatments are mainly performed in a spa or medical office. While some are actually "cross-over" treatments, meaning they can be done professionally or at home, I included them here as professional services that provide optimal results. I did not include a "Solution" section as these treatments are best left to the professionals to inform you how they're done. However, the description of the treatment provides an in-depth overview of the treatment, why it's done and what you can expect.

Spa Treatments

Microneedling

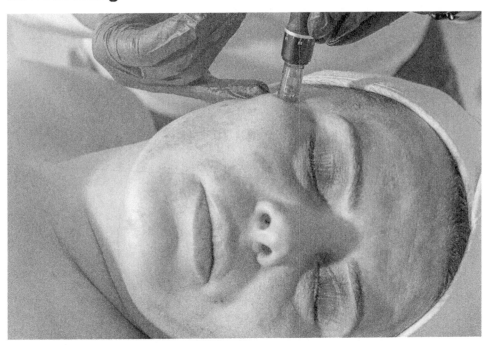

It's no secret that as we age our skin changes. Collagen production declines resulting in sagging and dullness, and the skin may appear looser with an uneven tone. We may get odd blemishes we've never seen or even develop rosacea. Our skin condition is often a reflection of our inner health, but the appearance may also be a matter of genes, scarring, or other trauma. Thankfully, science has found a way that we can reverse the clock a bit, through a procedure called microneedling.

Microneedling is commonly performed by a professional dermatologist or beautician. It is also called collagen induction therapy and is a procedure in which a device uses tiny needles to puncture the top layer of skin. The micro trauma prompts your skin to heal and rebuild itself, and it does so by synthesizing collagen and growth factors to build new tissue. Some known benefits are:

- Reverse or heal sun damage

- Lessen fine lines and wrinkles

- Treat scar damage

- Fight stretch marks

- Even out skin tone

- Improve skin's ability to hydrate (for plumpness)

Microneedling is a treatment best performed by a professional. They use a device that quickly injects tiny needles into the skin for a quick treatment. In some cases, your professional might use a topical anesthetic to reduce any pain. During the treatment various serums or even plasma can be used to penetrate into the skin and make the treatment even more effective and long lasting. Usually a mask is applied after the treatment to ensure healthy healing takes place while reducing or eliminating the chance for an infection.

A similar treatment can be performed at home, with a device called a "dermaroller." This is a cheaper alternative to salon treatments, but it can also be very effective. The dermaroller comes with tiny needles of various depths that you roll on your face or problem areas like a little wheel. Fine lines, acne scars, stretch marks and hyperpigmentation are all said to be reduced with regular derma rolling. It can also be used on the scalp to stimulate hair growth. With home use, you must be careful to properly disinfect your dermaroller after each treatment to avoid infections. You also need to make sure that the serums you're using are made specifically for this purpose.

A 2008 study found that four microneedling sessions resulted in up to a 400 percent rise in collagen, a protein that makes skin firmer.

Please make sure you get a good quality dermaroller, as with the cheaper imitation you can actually do a lot of harm to your skin. See this video for more info:

Channel: Gin Amber
Shocking truth about DERMAROLLERS, under the microscope

By cleansing your body on a regular basis and eliminating as many toxins as possible from your environment, your body can begin to heal itself, prevent disease, and become stronger and more resilient than you ever dreamed possible!

—Dr. Edward

Platelet Rich Plasma for Facial Rejuvenation

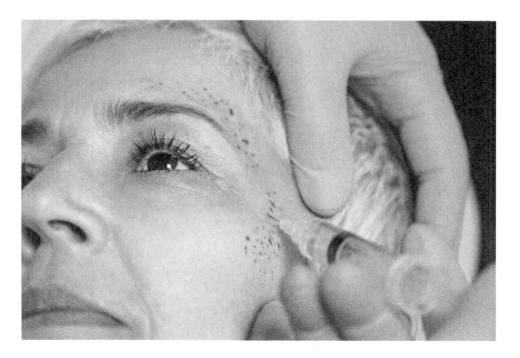

Platelet Rich Plasma (PRP) treatments refer to using PRP in combination with microneedling. The treatment gained popularity when celebrities around the world began posting photos of themselves getting the facial, which quickly became dubbed the vampire facial, as it looks as if one has blood smeared on the face.

In reality, this blood is plasma that is taken from your own arm. The plasma is then placed into a centrifuge machine where the platelets are separated from the blood. The leftover plasma is the solution that is used for the facial and is rich in growth factors that stimulate growth, in this case, growth of new skin cells. But they are also messengers that instruct skin cells to function, so that collagen and elastin are synthesized and utilized properly.

During a microneedling PRP treatment, your blood is drawn and then you will receive a microneedling treatment. As explained above, you will be left with many pinpoint sized holes in which serums can penetrate deeply into your skin. In this case, the serum is your plasma, or PRP. Some doctors prefer to inject PRP with a needle, instead of microneedling for a deeper and more lasting effect. The benefits of using PRP with are as follows:

A variety of PRP treatments exist, ranging from PRP treatment for joint and tendon pain and sports-related injuries, to cosmetic procedures used for anti-aging.

- Tighten and tone the skin

- Reduce fine lines and wrinkles

- Stimulates collagen production for volume

- Shrink large pores

- Smooth skin's texture

- Brighten skin tone and improve the quality

- Reduce acne scars

It should be noted that the benefits cannot be recreated by any other products because the PRP takes advantage of your body's own cells to create new and healthy skin. The entire process takes about 60 minutes and you will continue to see improvement in your skin for the next 2-3 months.

It is recommended that you do a treatment once a month for 3 months and then repeat once or twice a year. Doctors can also mix your plasma with collagen or hyaluronic acid for even better results.

Please see my video for more info:

Channel: The Aging Games
Vampire Facial (Before & After) ⏹ Platelet
Rich Plasma Facelift

PRP for Hair Loss

Platelet Rich Plasma (PRP) has been shown to help with hair growth as well. It is rich in growth factors that stimulate hair follicle activity, resulting in new hair growth. This is exciting for both men and women who are experiencing thinning hair and would prefer to avoid wigs, toupees or the more invasive hair transplants or plugs. Using your body's own cells to stimulate new growth anywhere is a healthy treatment that helps slow the aging process.

This procedure is performed by following the same steps as above; your blood is drawn and put into a centrifuge where the plasma is separated from the blood. Your physician will then inject the PRP into the scalp in an even pattern where it is needed. Cooling jets may be used to reduce inflammation and anesthetic may be used for comfort. And while it sounds extensive, the entire procedure often takes no longer than 30 minutes.

While PRP may not help you grow an entirely new head of hair, you should see improvement in fullness and thickness of your hair. In addition, you will experience less hair loss, so the results are compounded. It is best to start this treatment as soon as you start experiencing hair loss or

12 clinical trials were analyzed for the effectiveness of Platelet Rich Plasma in the treatment of Androgenetic Alopecia. In total, 84% of the studies (10 of 12) reported a positive effect of PRP for Androgenetic Alopecia treatment.

thinning, as it will be much more effective than for someone who lost their hair decades ago.

As for the face, 3 treatments are recommended 1 month apart and then repeated once or twice a year. You can use different products at home between treatments to keep the effects longer.

Please see my video for more info:

Channel: The Aging Games
Stop Hair Loss with Platelet Rich Plasma PRP | Does it work?

Get Regular Massages

Massage is more than a relaxing way to ward off stress. It has many therapeutic effects that are beneficial for both your body and your mind. While many of us think of massage as a luxury to be done once in a while, regular massages have full health benefits, many of which are anti-aging.

Massage is beneficial for both the face and the body. Facial massage brings more blood to the face, and the increased circulation naturally brings more oxygen and nutrients that support your body's ability to make collagen and elastin. The extra blood also gives your skin a beautiful glow, while helping to reduce congestion. During a facial massage lymphatic vessels are stimulated so more toxins are cleared out of the skin tissue, thus reducing puffiness. And lastly, massag-

Health is a relationship between you and your body

—Terri Guillemets

ing your face can help reduce stress and anxiety resulting in a more relaxed, youthful appearance.

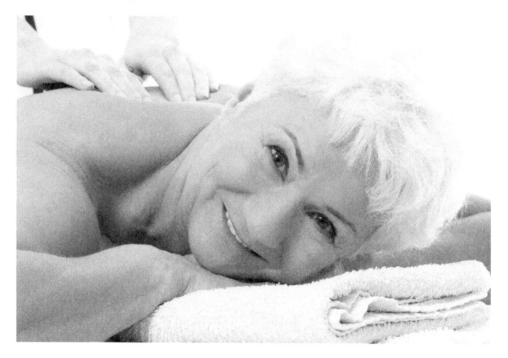

Full body massages also provide stress relief. Remember that stress produces an excess of certain hormones along with metabolic waste that can accelerate the aging process. A massage helps relax the muscles, making it easier to let go of stress and anxiety. At the same time, a full body massage lessens production of the stress hormone cortisol and increases the feel-good hormone, serotonin and relaxing hormone dopamine. This can result in better sleep and overall better disposition.

Massages increase production of oxytocin. Oxytocin is known as the "love hormone" because it is stimulated during hugging, cuddling and sex. Higher blood levels of oxytocin not only increase feelings of bonding, but have physical effects, as well. When oxytocin levels are low, muscles atrophy, or shrink at a quicker rate. And studies show that when the circulatory system is stimulated and hormones like oxytocin are increased, the regenerative capacity of our skeletal system can be improved. Since oxytocin production declines as we get older, regular massage can counter this. More oxytocin in our blood will not only save our muscles and bones from age-related deterioration, but we will also benefit from improved emotional health.

Massages stimulate blood flow, giving you a radiant glow while firming the skin.

Improved posture is another benefit of having regular massages. The rubbing action helps work out muscle tension and "stress bundle" where muscles tighten in a group. These can literally pull your spine out of place resulting in poor posture, which can have a negative effect on your circulation, digestion and nervous system. Regular massage trains the muscles to remain relaxed, making it easier to stand up straight while reducing back pain.

Earlier I mentioned how the lymphatic system relies on muscular contractions or manipulation for movement. It just so happens that massage is a way to manipulate muscles and help promote lymphatic drainage. This is especially important when we get older because our immune response naturally slows. Regular massage can counteract this effect as lymph is stimulated, increasing immune response.

Most spas and massage therapists provide discounts if you pay for a series of massages. If you are looking for a more economical way to take advantage of this amazing therapy, some massage schools offer free or very discounted services, as their students need to rack up a certain number of hours before they can get their license. And still another idea is to take lessons in therapeutic massage with a partner or spouse, and practice on each other. Try to get weekly massages or even biweekly, the more you can fit into your life, the happier you will feel.

Hyaluronic Acid

Hyaluronic acid (HA) is touted as an effective skin care ingredient to help plump the skin for a more youthful and fresher look. But hyaluronic acid is really a sugar molecule, or polysaccharide, that is a natural part of our skin and it helps bind collagen and water, which keeps collagen active in the skin. In appearance, it is a viscous, clear substance that our bodies naturally produce and most of it is found in the skin, eyes and our connective tissues.

Time And health are two precious assets that we don't recognize and appreciate until they have been depleted.

—Denis Waitley

As our bodies mature, the ability to produce HA lessens and our skin ages with less ability to hold moisture. Collagen and elastin production degrade, and our skin begins to show the signs of aging as it sags and thins. Once again, technology comes to the rescue with topical and injectable forms of HA for a cosmetic anti-aging solution.

Hyaluronic acid has been shown to be beneficial in many uses. As a supplement, research found that the body does distribute HA to connective tissue.[1] HA is also beneficial when applied topically for skin hydration and via injection to effectively treat wrinkles. Because it is an ingredient

---

1 Balogh L, Polyak A, Mathe D, Kiraly R, Thuroczy J, Terez M, Janoki G, Ting Y, Bucci LR, Schauss AG. Absorption, uptake and tissue affinity of high-molecular-weight hyaluronan after oral administration in rats and dogs. J Agric Food Chem. 2008 Nov 26;56(22):10582-93. doi: 10.1021/jf8017029. PMID: 18959406.

that is natural to the body, there are few side effects (pregnant women and those with cancer should avoid it).

Benefits of HA are numerous, which is why it remains a popular treatment today. When applied topically, it acts as a humectant, as it attracts water and holds it to the skin, keeping it plump and fresh looking. Added hydration with increased plumpness helps reduce fine lines, resulting in healthier and more youthful looking skin. And it is interesting to note that HA is also used to help accelerate healing of skin injuries like wounds and scars.

In cosmetic dermatology, HA is used as a dermal filler to add volume and reduce wrinkles, facial folds and fine lines. It is also used to add volume in facial areas that may need it and to naturally plump lips, so they are fuller and more youthful. Added plumpness in the lips also reduces the fine lines that can gather around the mouth as we age.

For sure we've all seen some very bad examples of lip fillers when it's overdone so when it comes to using fillers, moderation is key. There is a fine line between using a well-placed HA filler to balance the face and overfilling lips and cheeks, leading to that pillow-face you see many celebrities sporting. Also keep in mind that overfilling the face can actually stretch out the skin and lead to more sagging, especially in the jowl area. If you do decide to get HA fillers, please go to a reputable doctor whose work you have seen. The best type of filler will slightly enhance your face without anyone even noticing. Most fillers today last between 6-18 months.

Hyaluronic acid can enhance moisture content beyond comparison. It also revitalizes skin's surface layers, making it softer, smoother and radiantly hydrated. This instantly improves the appearance of fine lines and wrinkles.

The HA found in serums, creams and injectables may come from the comb of a rooster or from a plant-based product that contains wheat. But the main source of HA is through microbial fermentation, which is a natural way to produce this type of polysaccharide. This method is also more cost-effective and eco-friendlier, but learn the source before you use it in case you have allergies.

Retinol Skin Care

Retinol is one of the most powerful derivatives of vitamin A that is used in dermatology to promote collagen synthesis, brighten the skin and even the skin tone. It is one of the most studied of all retinoids (vitamin A derivatives), making it one of the most popular ingredients used in anti-aging beauty products. The best part is that it does not only work cosmetically, but also works as an antioxidant that can lessen the damage done to the skin by free radicals, which are a major cause of premature aging.

One of the ways retinol works is by accelerating skin cell turnover, which essentially tricks your body into treating your skin as if it were younger. When cell turnover is increased, you can enjoy a consistently new supply of fresh skin cells on the skin's surface, which helps reduce fine lines and improves your skin's texture. Your skin tone will also even out as older, sun damaged cells are removed on a deeper level, eventually removing and replacing them with fresh, new cells.

When searching for anti-aging skin care products, look for either retinyl palmitate if you have very dry or sensitive skin, or the stronger and still tolerable retinol. If you are unsure, ask your dermatologist or beautician which version is best for you.

Once you do find a product, begin your retinol skin care regimen slowly. The following tips can help:

- Choose the right strength; retinyl palmitate for sensitive skin, retinol or retinaldehyde for normal skin or adapalene for acne-prone skin.

- Do not use retinol products with any other skin care products until you have acclimated your skin to them and are certain you have no allergies.

- Do not use with another facial peel or acid.

- Begin very slowly with a pea-sized drop, once a week at first, then move up to twice and then three times each week. Your specific products might have their own instructions, so it is best to follow those closely or even more slowly.

- Be careful with the sun when you first get started as Retinol can temporarily make your skin more sensitive to the sun.

Eliminate Age Spots

Age spots are small dark areas found anywhere on the skin including the face, hands and arms. Also known as liver spots, as the state of our skin can be directly related to our liver's ability to detoxify, although some experts now argue that the liver doesn't have anything to do with age spots. However, our skin is the largest organ of our body and is a reflection 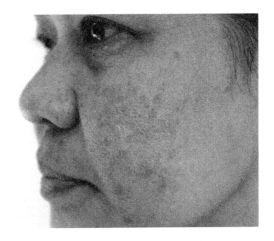 of our internal health. When our liver does not function well or if we lack the extra nutrition that we need as we get older, then it will be reflected on our skin. Hormonal issues, such as excess estrogen, can also be a contributing factor.

The most obvious culprit in the appearance of dark pigmentation is the sun, but this doesn't really tell the whole story. You might be surprised to learn that what you're eating will play a large role in how your skin reacts to the UV rays from sunlight. Research by Dr Ray Peat suggests that the right diet is crucial in age spot prevention. The sun isn't actually the source of skin aging either; it only contributes to skin damage with overexposure and when a person has accumulated too much PUFA (Polyunsaturated fatty acids from canola, soy, corn, safflower, and sunflower oils) in their tissues.

If you don't take time to take care of your health now, you're gonna have to make time for feeling sick and tired later.

—Karen Salmansohn

"While it is important to avoid overexposure to ultraviolet light, the skin damage that we identify with aging is largely a product of our diet," says Dr. Peat. "I am convinced that replacing PUFAs with saturated fats is the best thing you can do for both your skin and body."

The bad news is that it takes four years to fully detoxify PUFAs from your tissues, but gradually you should notice an improvement in your metabolism and fewer age spots, among other benefits.

What can you do in the meantime?

The first step is to cleanse and detoxify your body with a liver flush by following the instructions in the section on how to remove gallbladder and liver stones. The liver is connected to the gallbladder, and will actually fill up with stones before the gallbladder gets overburdened, according to Andreas Moritz, the author of The Amazing Liver Cleanse.

Attack age spots from the outside with these remedies:

- Exfoliate with papaya to remove dead skin cells, increase collage production and allow topical remedies to better penetrate.

If you don't take time to take care of your health now, you're gonna have to make time for feeling sick and tired later.

—Karen Salmansohn

- Make a mask with equal parts turmeric and honey. Add a couple of drops of lemon juice or lemon essential oil and apply to the age spots and allow to sit for 20 to 30 minutes before washing off.

- Creams and serums with lemon oil and bearberry are effective for fading age spots.

- Talk to your dermatologist about hydroquinone, a prescription cream to remove age spots.

- Professional chemical peels have been effectively used to lighten age spots.

- Laser treatments are very effective. The treatment is performed by a professional dermatologist or cosmetic physician, but can quickly remove age spots with results lasting longer than creams.

- Intense Pulsed Light (IPL) is a professional treatment that uses a broadband light source as opposed to the monochromatic of a laser. During the procedure you are given dark glasses and a cooling gel is applied to the face, then light pulses will be directed at the skin. This treatment is also known as a photofacial and can treat many skin conditions at the same time.

According to Dr. Ray Peat, "brown pigment that generally increases with age, and its formation is increased by consumption of unsaturated fats, by vitamin E deficiency, by stress, and by exposure to excess estrogen."

Please keep in mind that these are all superficial solutions and will not give permanent results until the underlying issues are addressed.

HIFU Facials

A High Intensity Focused Ultrasound Facial, or HIFU facial uses ultrasound to heat and damage cells deep in the skin to stimulate a healing response in the skin with increased collagen production. The result is as close as one can get to a face lift without undergoing surgery.

In 2009, the Food and Drug Administration (FDA) approved HIFU for brow lifts, then later on cleared the treatment to treat wrinkles as well. FDA clearing means the procedure showed enough evidence that it was effective enough to make these claims, so you can be sure you will see results when you get this treatment. Please keep in mind that there are huge differences in HIFU machines and the highest strength will only be available at a medical spa or doctor's office. You also need to be very careful as in the wrong hands and with the wrong machine, you can actually be melting fat in parts of your face where you might not want to.

The following are the benefits that patients expect with a HIFU facial:

• Skin tightening on neck

• Less wrinkles

• Enhanced definition of the jawline

- Eyebrow, eyelid and cheek lift

- Smoother skin

- Reduction in double chin

The HIFU facial provides more natural results since it stimulates the body to create its own collagen and repair. It is said to have a 94% efficacy, or improvement, without the harsh side effects or risk that surgery might have. There is also no downtime, since the machine only sends heat deep into the dermis, while leaving the top layer of your skin undisturbed. HIFU can also safely be used on different parts of the body, such as the arms, stomach and buttocks.

The procedure is similar to other beauty treatments, and this is what you can expect during a session:

- Your face (or area to be treated) will be cleansed

- Topical anesthetic may be applied, followed by ultrasound gel

- The HIFU device is placed against your skin and adjusted by the physician

- Ultrasound energy is delivered to your face (lasting 30-60 mins)

- You may feel heat or tingling like pin pricks

You will see optimal results about 3 months after your treatment and it's recommended to have touch-ups about once a year.

HIFU is used by leading medical clinics and you can expect results to last between 12-18 months from a single session.

Please check out my video about HIFU:

Channel: The Aging Games
Ultraformer 3 HIFU (High Intensity Focused Ultrasound)
Body Treatment | My Experience

Radiofrequency for Tighter Skin

Radiofrequency (RF) is the use of energy waves to cause molecular friction, which heats the area and contracts collagen fibers. The result is an immediate lift to the skin for a tightening effect. At the same time, the treatment stimulates collagen synthesis, so the benefits are twofold.

Studies show that heating the skin to a certain temperature creates something called heat-shock proteins, which produce a cumulative healing effect.[2] This leads to the synthesis of new elastin and collagen fibers, which creates the network that helps keep skin firm. These effects also lead to other benefits such as:

* Improvements to sun damaged skin

* Body contouring as it lifts skin in all areas including the thighs, stomach and upper arms

* Face contouring and face slimming

* Minimizing under-eye wrinkles

The procedure is relatively painless with minimal side effects like redness and possible swelling. Because each skin type is different, your cosmetic physician or dermatologist can determine the depth of RF waves to use.

2   Rousseaux I, Robson S. Body Contouring and Skin Tightening Using a Unique Novel Multisource Radiofrequency Energy Delivery Method. J Clin Aesthet Dermatol. 2017;10(4):24-29.

It is recommended that you do a series of weekly sessions for optimal results.

A newer, more powerful treatment is RF Microneedling for skin tightening, collagen remodeling (production and healthy connections) and overall skin rejuvenation. In this case, the dermatologist uses a special device with special needles that deliver high-intensity radio frequency energy during the microneedling treatment. This is a more invasive treatment that will probably require local anesthetic and a longer downtime but the results will also be more visible and longer lasting.

I've included radiofrequency treatments in this book because I have used these treatments successfully myself, however, please do keep in mind that it does involve a low form of radiation so please do your research to determine if this treatment is right for you. The RF energy used in skin tightening is in the range of 450 KHz, which is on the very low end of the spectrum. To put it into perspective, according to Healthline, the form of radiation used in RF skin tightening releases about 1 billion times less energy than X-rays.

With radiofrequency, the skin is heated at a more superficial level to trigger collagen production. There's really little to no downtime.

Stem Cell Facelift

In the past decade, Stem Cell Facelifts have become very popular as a safer alternative to traditional facelifts. As with the PRP treatment, this therapy uses the healing and rejuvenating power of your own cells, but in the form of stem

"

Your health is what you make of it. Everything you do and think either adds to the vitality, energy, and spirit you possess or takes away from it.

—Ann Wigmore

The stem cells that are injected into the face will mimic and help stimulate the cells around them, facilitating and encouraging a natural healing and rejuvenating processes to take place.

cells this time, derived from your own adipose tissue (fat tissue).

This method is more invasive than PRP as actual surgery is required to remove the adipose tissue through liposuction. This is not a large amount and can be performed with just local anesthetic. The fat will then be processed to separate the stem cells, and these stem cells are what will be injected into your facial tissues. If you have lost a lot of facial volume or in place of fillers, they can also reinject some of your own fat where needed. This procedure restores the volume of the face, while the stem cells will work to texture and tone, thus producing smoother, younger-looking skin.

Benefits of a Stem Cell Facelift include:

• Stimulates your own collagen production

• Restores facial volume

• Enhances jawline definition

• Produces natural and long-lasting results

• Faster recovery with minimal scarring

Please keep in mind that while a Stem Cell Facelift can bring about great improvements, if you have a lot of loose skin, it might not give you enough tightening to give you the results you're looking for.

Fat transfer with stem cells is also being used today for breast enhancement and for the famous Brazilian Butt Lift.

Medical Treatments

Bioidentical Hormone Therapy (BHRT)

As we get older, it is natural for hormones to decline in production along with a host of other biological changes. Hormone replacement therapy has been the standing treatment for menopausal women, testosterone decline in men, endocrine therapy and possibly as part of a comprehensive cancer treatment.

Imbalanced hormones can lead to not only symptoms that interfere with the quality of life (like hot flashes and vaginal dryness), but also to possible health issues. Some symptoms that may be due to hormonal imbalances include:

- Depression or anxiety
- Fatigue
- Hair loss
- Memory loss
- Mood changes
- Sleep disturbances
- Increased body fat, especially around the middle
- Decreased libido
- Pain during intercourse
- Erectile issues

According to Dr. Josh Axe, certified doctor of natural medicine and clinical nutritionist, some specific problems are associated with some of the most common hormonal imbalances, including:

Estrogen dominance: changes in sleep patterns, changes in weight and appetite, higher perceived stress, slowed metabolism

Polycystic Ovarian Syndrome (PCOS): infertility, weight gain, higher risk for diabetes, acne, abnormal hair growth

The goal of BHRT is to restore youthful hormone levels in a way that safely and effectively combats symptoms of aging and related diseases. Ideal hormone levels are essential for peak health in both men and women as we age.

Low estrogen: low sex drive, reproductive problems, menstrual irregularity, changes in mood

Hypothyroidism: slowed metabolism, weight gain, fatigue, anxiety, irritability, digestive issues, irregular periods

Low testosterone: erectile dysfunction, muscle loss, weight gain, fatigue, mood-related problems

Hyperthyroidism & Grave's disease: anxiety, thinning hair, weight loss, IBS, trouble sleeping, irregular heartbeats

Diabetes: weight gain, nerve damage (neuropathy), higher risk for vision loss, fatigue, trouble breathing, dry mouth, skin problems

Adrenal fatigue: fatigue, muscle aches and pains, anxiety and depression, trouble sleeping, brain fog, reproductive problems

Getting the appropriate treatment for your hormonal health can help you live a higher quality of life and remain healthy well into your later decades. And along with these benefits, hormone therapy can actually slow down the aging process.

Due to the side effects of synthetic Hormone Replacement Therapy (HRT) which are often derived from animals (for example from horse urine), scientists have created bioidentical hormones, which are synthesized from plants. Bioidentical hormones identically match the structure of our human hormones, so it's a far more natural approach to hormone therapy. There are some very interesting books on the topic, especially by Suzanne Somers, who looks amazing at 74 and has done tremendous research in this area.

If you do decide to try Bioidentical Hormones, make sure you find a physician who specializes in this field. Balancing hormones is a very difficult undertaking and you need to know all the risks involved.

There are also some natural ways you can balance your hormones yourself and some of these include:

- Cold Therapy

- Red Light Therapy

- Dietary changes

- Removing toxic chemicals from your food and environment

- Managing stress (through regular medication for example)

- Making sure you're getting enough sleep

- Reducing inflammation

- Using essential oils

- Using herbal supplements

Low-Dose Naltrexone

Naltrexone is a medication that was originally used to help people addicted to opium and heroin in order to

LDN is a little known yet life-changing medication with more and more success stories in the Functional Medicine world. It may just be the magic pill for those with autoimmune conditions and difficulty losing weight.

stop drug use. It was found that this drug consists of an equal part of two isomers, or shapes. One shape binds to opioid receptors, which can help remove the craving for opioids associated with addiction, while the other shape of naltrexone binds to immune cells. In other words, the two isomers have different biological activity, making this an effective medication that supports your immune system.

While high dosage Naltrexone (50—100 mg/day) appears to negate the immune effect, low dose Naltrexone (.05—3 mg/day) is effective at the following:

- Stimulates the release of endorphins

- Endorphins help modulate immune response

- Inhibits the growth of unwanted, or harmful cells

- Inhibits cytokine, which can suppress immunity

- Reduces pain and inflammation

- Fights many different kinds of cancer

- Often used for autoimmune conditions such as Hashimoto's, fibromyalgia, arthritis, and MS

Low dose Naltrexone (LDN) is identical to an endorphin which is natural to the body. This is the mechanism that stops the inflammatory response that causes pain and destruction of tissue. It also seems to protect nerve cells from damage and degeneration, and supports brain cells. Today, many use it as a form of protection from age-related, autoimmune diseases and cancer.

Many doctors still don't have any knowledge of LDN so in order to get a prescription you'd have to search out a physician who likely specializes in alternative therapies. LDN has been proven to be a safe and non-addictive therapy and a life saver for many, especially for those suffering from autoimmune conditions. There are many support groups on Facebook where you can read about personal stories from people who have been taking it for a while.

Biofeedback and Heart Rate Variability

Heart rate is regulated by the sympathetic and parasympathetic branches of the autonomic nervous system (ANS). The interaction of the two branches are responsible for various systems like the cardiovascular, digestive and endocrine systems to help us respond to a changing environment.

Heart rate variability (HRV) measures the pause between heartbeats and high HRV is associated with reduced mortality and good health. The pause between heartbeats is not "regular" or consistent, but should change throughout the day. This is an indication that one can adapt more easily and is associated with good physical and psychological health. But low HRV seems to be related to a stressed state, causing the body to become stuck in the "fight" side of "fight or flight." We know this as chronic stress and it can interfere with everything from mental health to digestion, as well as accelerated aging and early death.

While HRV can be measured with Smartwatch apps and similar tools, biofeedback can not only measure but help you improve your HRV biomarker. With an improved HRV, you are more in control of slowing the aging process within yourself thanks to these benefits:

The doctor of the future will no longer treat the human frame with drugs, but rather will cure and prevent disease with nutrition.

—**Thomas Edison**

There now is a unique, high-tech method called Beauty Biofeedback, which helps reduce stress and trains the cells of your face and body to regenerate for a more youthful appearance.

- Lowered blood pressure as you train yourself to relax at will, and lower blood pressure lowers your risk for heart disease

- Deeper and more rejuvenating sleep as a result from a healthier nervous system

- Reduced cortisol levels: cortisol is the stress hormone that can lead to heart disease, digestive problems and insomnia, but improved HRV means you can recover from stress and move on

- Remain in control of your body, thoughts and emotions as you train yourself to better handle stress with biofeedback

Fortunately, modern technology has allowed us to learn how to use biofeedback to improve HRV right in our own homes. Online courses teach how to manage stress using breathing exercises and other tools to improve vagal tone and manage stress. Ultimately, the goal is to learn resilience, which means you will be in control of how you react to and let go of stress. The result is improved emotional and physical health.

The Importance of Sex

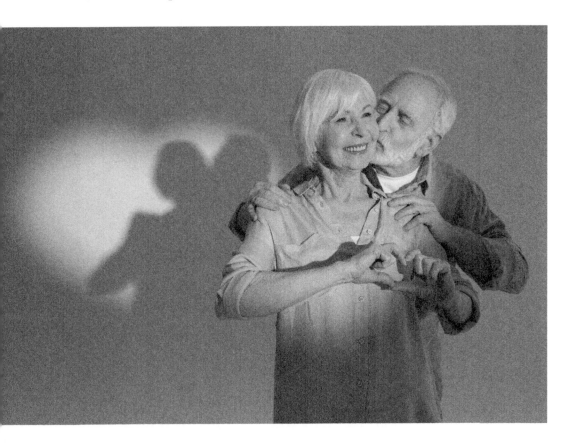

Having sex promotes improved mental and physical health. When we lose our sexuality, we also lose a valuable aspect of ourselves. Our sexual self builds confidence and helps us connect with our bodies. It is a way to express love for another and strengthen an emotional connection. And when we lose our desire for sex, it could be an indication of an underlying health issue and hormonal imbalances.

Most people don't realize that regular sex is very important for healthy hormonal function. In fact, it stimulates the release of both estrogen and testosterone, which are anti-aging hormones. Estrogen promotes healthy

Physical issues that can cause low libido include low testosterone, prescription medicines, too little or too much exercise, and alcohol and drug use. Psychological issues can include depression, stress, and problems in your relationship.

skin and hair, while testosterone is necessary for strong bones, a healthy heart, good muscle tone and the ability to lose fat. Even better, the estrogen released during sex promotes the formation of collagen for firm skin.

The period just before orgasm promotes a surge of endorphins and release of the love hormone, oxytocin. These are natural pain reducers, and both promote better mental health. Endorphins are also known to improve the immune system and research has found that those who have regular sex also have higher levels of Immunoglobulin A, which protects you from infection.

If you suffer from lack of a sex drive, it might be signs of depression, chronic stress or hormonal imbalances, all of which contribute to a lesser quality of life. But quality of life becomes even more important as we age, so taking care of your health, including sexual health, can benefit other areas of your life. As we have seen, each of these factors can lead to physical health problems like heart disease and cancer. Chronic stress, depression and hormonal imbalances can also accelerate the aging process and make us look older.

If you have issues with your libido, try some of the things mentioned in this book or see your doctor. If you prefer to use natural methods, seek out a Naturopathic Doctor who specializes in hormonal health or an acupuncturist or other natural health practitioner. There are numerous ways to get help, and with a little effort you will be sure to find one that resonates with you.

Natural ways to increase libido are very similar to the ones I mentioned for balancing hormones and improving overall health will also go a long way.

Check out my video on how to increase Testosterone naturally, a very important hormone for both men and women:

Health is like money, we never have a true idea of its value until we lose it.

—Josh Billings

Channel: The Aging Games
How to Increase Testosterone Levels Naturally

Vaginal Rejuvenation

Vaginal rejuvenation is a term to describe the tightening and strengthening of the vaginal walls. Hormonal changes, age, and childbirth all contribute to vaginal laxity, which also results in loss of lubrication, urinary incontinence and pain during sex. But rejuvenation in this area can help incontinence, build self-esteem, improve collagen production and increase pleasure during sex.

Vaginal rejuvenation improves vaginal laxity and can be done in a number of ways. Some of these are as follows:

• Kegel exercises are widely used by many for tightening vaginal muscles. Begin by stopping urination in midstream to identify your pelvic muscles. Next focus on those muscles, tighten and hold them for 10 seconds, and repeat 10 to 15 times, three times a day. Some people teach to imagine sitting on a marble and then picking it up with your pelvic floor muscles.

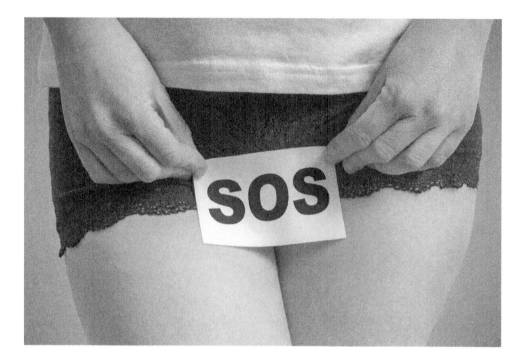

- Kegel weights take the above exercises to the next level. They were recommended by the original creator of the Kegel exercises and can improve your results.

- Yoni eggs are a way to mimic Kegel exercises but with a tangible item instead of the imagination. The goal of exercising with a yoni egg is to strengthen the pelvic floor, which results in more toned muscles, increase control of the urinary tract to avoid incontinence, improved lubrication and improved sensation in the vaginal canal.

- Ben-wa balls are similar in how they exercise vaginal walls. They are often a series of two or more balls connected by a string, which are then inserted into the vagina. Some advocate wearing them inside as you go about the day, but exercises can be found that are intended to directly strengthen the pelvic floor.

- Jumping on a mini trampoline can help build strengthen and tighten your pelvic floor muscles along with all the other supportive muscles in your entire abdominal area. Begin with only 2 minutes of jumping and work your way up to 10 or 20 minutes each day.

- Laser and RF energy are non-surgical options to improve sexual function and vaginal laxity. In both cases, a device is used in a professional setting to heat the area and increase collagen production. This method costs more than doing your own work at home, but can give quicker results.

Nearly 50% of menopausal women complain of vaginal dryness, itching, and burning, among other commonly reported menopausal symptoms.

The doctor of the future will no longer treat the human frame with drugs, but rather will cure and prevent disease with nutrition.

—Thomas Edison

CHAPTER 8

Additional Links & Resources

My friend, Jason Christoff, has developed a worldwide reputation as a self-sabotage coach who makes complex issues easy to understand for his clients.

A Healthy Living Guide with Linked Educational Sources

The primary benefit for reducing toxins and insults to the body, is in regard to the resulting stress and inflammation that all of these factors inflict on the metabolism plus the changes in body shape/brain function that this stress/inflammation cycle can initiate. Gaining weight and in-flammation through non-calorie insults and general stress is called environmental weight gain. **https://bit.ly/2HYwl0Y**

By reducing and eliminating the cause of inflammation and stress within your daily habits… diseases can lift, weight can be lost, water retention reduced, cellulite genesis halted, and all matters of health, vitality and strength increased. It's never about "adding on" complex solutions. It's always about "removing" what's already hurting us and then walking effortlessly into a better way of being. The below listed factors are greatly involved in aggravating the body and causing its breakdown. Simply stop or reduce the aggravating factors and replace those with modalities that heal or that are proven benign. Let this list guide you quickly toward all your success-based goals. Please remember as well that a polluted mind can't think properly, so this isn't just about the physical. Cleaning up is about the mental, the physical, the spiritual plus the financial as well. You can only succeed on all levels if your mind, body and spirit are clean. An unhealthy body is always coupled with a dysfunctional and unhealthy mind (and mind set). The toxic modality (that you want to remove) is listed first with each point… and healing modality (that you want to implement) is listed second. Enjoy…

1. Teflon Pans (stainless steel) – https://bit.ly/2VjJ6ko – The Devil We Know – Documentary on The Extreme Dangers of Teflon

2. Plastic Food Containers (glass) https://bit.ly/2VfFKPf

3. Mercury Fillings (white resin)… remove mercury fillings at dentist certified by https://iaomt.org only (Documentary

4. Evidence of Harm Trailer https://bit.ly/2HQb13j and the German documentary QueckSilbder https://bit.ly/3c4Jf12)

5. All Medications – Prescription and Over the Counter (get healthy – reduce or eliminate all medications) – medications and the medical system are the #1 cause of premature death in the United States and the EU https://bit.ly/39YKzAw – video from medical doctor Dr. Jospeh Mercola and book by medical doctor Dr. Carolyn Dean and Gary Null medical researcher and PhD – https://bit.ly/38UiMkA

6. Cell Phones (away at least 3 feet, hands free, airplane mode) – many cited resources in one document from Jason Christoff - https://bit.ly/2v3nLRx

7. Cordless Phones (corded phones) – the same threat applies to cordless phones as to cell phones plus wireless routers, ear buds, smart watches, fit bits, baby monitors, blue tooth, wireless speakers and any cordless wireless device etc – the best author in this field is Nick Penault and his latest book – https://bit.ly/2TcLEhl

8. Wireless Routers (wireless off before bed, hard line the router as soon as possible, when you hard wire the router, make sure your computer wifi is also off) – same article from Jason Christoff on the dangers of wireless devices – https://bit.ly/2v3nLRx

9. Smart TV's (remove microwave emitting device) – here's some instructions for turning the Wi-Fi emitter off if that's a possibility

https://youtu.be/bnW1_hM3iO8 and here are some instructions for removing it from the TV altogether – https://youtu.be/skfDt-N63XD4 – I personally would hire an audio/video specialist at a computer/TV store to remove this for me

10. Living Too Close To Power Lines (think about making a move) – both large open area power lines https://bit.ly/2SZfuXM and thicker neighborhood power lines are an issue https://bit.ly/2w10Xlw

11. Staying Up Past 10:30 (go to bed by 10 pm) https://rb.gy/juvb74

12. Getting Up Before the Sun – (get up with the sun) – same information as point 10. You need to sync to the cycles of the sun, regardless of season, to stay in optimal health.

13. Chemicals Common in Non Organic Processed Foods (eat more natural food) – https://bit.ly/2uqGNRg

14. Pesticides Common on Non Organic Produce (eat organic) – https://bit.ly/390Ntob and https://chem-tox.com/pesticides/

15. Pesticides and Chemicals Common in Non-Organic Meat (eat organic) https://bit.ly/3c42s2V

16. Genetically Modified Foods (use organic only, especially in the GMO food categories) https://bit.ly/2w6TgKk

17. Coffee – (reduce and quit eventually or quit right away) https://bit.ly/2HX4h3A

18. Pasteurized Commercial Fruit Juices (make your juice fresh) https://bit.ly/3c9EnYg

19. Sugar Based Energy Drinks Like Gatorade, Powerade (quit) https://bit.ly/3a53c5O

20. Caffeine Based Energy Drinks Like Red Bull, Rock Star etc (quit immediately) https://bit.ly/2SYShVG

21. Under Arm Deodorants with Aluminum (use aluminum free) – avoid all aluminum based products –https://bit.ly/2w8krEw)

22. Fluoride Tooth Pastes (use fluoride free) https://bit.ly/2PmULLg and https://bit.ly/2SZmcNs

23. Chocolate and Caffeine Based Teas (quit) – same as caffeine-based info above

24. Non-Organic Personal Care Products (start subbing in organic) – https://bit.ly/32pNVtO comic and accurate

25. All Alcohol (quit) – https://bit.ly/38GmWvL

26. Flavored Waters (drink only spring or natural sparkling) – https://bit.ly/2IxlgK9

27. Fabric Softener (quit or use natural options) – https://bit.ly/3ag7p75 softener falls in this category

28. Artificial Sweeteners (quit) (https://bit.ly/32tmoaJ and https://bit.ly/2PEsZKD)

29. Microwaved Food (destroy and recycle it) https://bit.ly/3a4dG5p

30. Wheat Gluten – wheat pizza, pasta, breads, bagels, pancakes, toast etc – (go organic and gluten free) https://bit.ly/2SWSrgk and https://bit.ly/2w3kXDV

31. Pasteurized Dairy (use unpasteurized organic or quit) https://bit.ly/2VoezSy and https://bit.ly/3a2AbYp

32. Toxic Conventional Sunscreens (use full spectrum non-toxic versions) https://bit.ly/2TeW7J5 and https://bit.ly/37UsoKN

33. Too Frequent and Too Intense Exercise (listen to your body) https://bit.ly/3a8f6vZ and https://bit.ly/38Z6FTB

34. Tattoos and Piercings (quit… everyone has them, they're not original) https://bit.ly/2HW2R9y and https://bit.ly/3a8VSq1 and https://bit.ly/3ci5MaK

35. Junk food, Candy, Sweets, Ice Cream, Pastries, Pies (quit) https://bit.ly/32xe6yL

36. Movie Theatre Popcorn Butter – huge cancer causer – (bring healthy snacks) https://bit.ly/2Psb4Xo

37. The Toxic Coating Inside All Take-Out Containers (don't pollute, protect your health as well… don't use them) https://bit.ly/2w9S4px and https://bit.ly/3c671JT

38. Stale and Uncirculated Air Inside the Home (open the windows often) https://cnb.cx/32BPJ3b

39. Elective Surgeries That Leave Foreign Objects Inside the Body (work on decorating the inside instead – love yourself as you are or explant) – https://bit.ly/32pC2EI

40. Non-Elective Surgeries That Remove Organs (live healthy, question the belief that you can be healthy without all your parts) https://www.hersfoundation.org/adverse-effects-data/

41. Stinkin Thinking – an addiction to crisis and chaos – (get healthy and the mind changes itself for the better) – https://bit.ly/38551yw

42. Chemical Perfumes, Fragrances and Sprays (sub in organic versions) – https://bit.ly/3c7mzgp

43. Toxic House Cleaning Supplies (sub in organic versions) – https://bit.ly/3ag7p75

44. Vaccines (educate before you vaccinate – many doctors don't vaccinate their own children or themselves... find out why) – many doctors and documentaries – https://bit.ly/2HXt4Vn

45. Aluminum Pans and Tin Foils (use steel-based cooking pots, and pans, the gold standard is sold from salad master https://salad-master.com/ and if in the US, Sadie King can service you directly Info@conscious-cook.com) https://bit.ly/2HRvfts

46. Chlorine in Tap Water and Swimming Pools (salt water pool to swim in, clean spring water to drink) https://bit.ly/393c5N6 – filter for shower head and bath https://bit.ly/2VikqbX and https://bit.ly/2HSvjcs

47. Conventional Table Salt (Himalayan sea salt) – https://bit.ly/32tbeml

48. Commercial Low-Quality Vitamins, Protein Powders, Supplements (use Innate Response or Mega Food Organic) – https://bit.ly/3c9WBJa

49. Margarine (use organic butter, ghee and coconut oil) – https://bit.ly/32u0aFA

50. Commercial Salad Dressings – that use soy, canola, corn, cottonseed, safflower or sunflower oils – https://bit.ly/32rMbQK (make your own with olive oil)

51. Smoking Marijuana (vaporize, ingest or quit) – https://bit.ly/3a5kPCE

52. Smoking Cigarettes (quit) – https://bit.ly/3826WDQ

53. Light from TV or Computer Screen After Sundown – (less screen time) – https://rb.gy/juvb74

54. Pop and Diet Pop (quit or get your affairs in order) https://bit.ly/2la37Cd and https://bit.ly/2wH4N3l

55. Junk Food and Fast Food (love and care for yourself to a higher standard) – https://bit.ly/37V1wuk and https://bit.ly/2Psbl79

56. Sunglasses – (don't wear them as much as possible or never wear sunglasses) – https://bit.ly/3aaCdWL

The reason these items cause weight gain, disease, brain damage, self-sabotage and cellulite etc., is because every one of these items are proven to stress the body. The stress system is the fat gain system. A body under stress increases fat gain and water retention in an attempt to dilute and buffer the toxic insult. Cortisol, a stress hormone, when in excess…. causes brain damage. A stressed body can't make optimal decisions as well because it's in a low IQ fight, flight or freeze mode of operation. Although one item on the list most often won't cause a massive amount of fat gain or disease on its' own, combining these toxic attacks (one on top of each other) can indeed trigger large increases in weight gain and sudden onset of chronic disease. Go over the list and see what items you can remove from your lifestyle, in an effort to accomplish your health and life success related goals.

To find out more or to contact Jason, please visit his website: https://jchristoff.com/about-us/

Printed in Great Britain
by Amazon

72317577R00147